Pain Management

Editors

JULIE G. PILITSIS
JOSHUA M. ROSENOW

NEUROSURGERY
CLINICS OF NORTH AMERICA

www.neurosurgery.theclinics.com

Consulting Editors
RUSSELL R. LONSER
DANIEL K. RESNICK

July 2022 • Volume 33 • Number 3

ELSEVIER

1600 John F. Kennedy Boulevard • Suite 1800 • Philadelphia, Pennsylvania, 19103-2899

http://www.theclinics.com

NEUROSURGERY CLINICS OF NORTH AMERICA Volume 33, Number 3
July 2022 ISSN 1042-3680, ISBN-13: 978-0-323-85017-9

Editor: Stacy Eastman
Developmental Editor: Ann Gielou Posedio

Neurosurgery Clinics of North America (ISSN 1042-3680) is published quarterly by Elsevier Inc., 360 Park Avenue South, New York, NY 10010-1710. Months of issue are January, April, July, and October. Business and Editorial Offices: 1600 John F. Kennedy Blvd., Suite 1800, Philadelphia, PA 19103-2899. Customer Service Office: 11830 Westline Industrial Drive, St. Louis, MO 63146. Periodicals postage paid at New York, NY, and additional mailing offices. Subscription prices are $447.00 per year (US individuals), $1,043.00 per year (US institutions), $479.00 per year (Canadian individuals), $1,074.00 per year (Canadian institutions), $556.00 per year (international individuals), $1,074.00 per year (international institutions), $100.00 per year (US students), $255.00 per year (international students), and $100.00 per year (Canadian students). International air speed delivery is included in all *Clinics* subscription prices. All prices are subject to change without notice. **POSTMASTER:** Send address changes to *Neurosurgery Clinics of North America*, Elsevier Periodicals Customer Service, 11830 Westline Industrial Drive, St. Louis, MO 63146. **Customer Service: 1-800-654-2452 (US and Canada). From outside the US and Canada, call: 1-314-453-7041. Fax: 1-314-453-5170. E-mail: JournalsCustomerService-usa@elsevier.com (for print support) and journalsonlinesupport-usa@elsevier.com (for online support).**

Reprints. For copies of 100 or more, of articles in this publication, please contact the Commercial Reprints Department, Elsevier Inc., 360 Park Avenue South, New York, NY 10010-1710. Tel. 212-633-3874; Fax: 212-633-3820; E-mail: reprints@elsevier.com.

Neurosurgery Clinics of North America is covered in *MEDLINE/PubMed (Index Medicus), EMBASE/Excerpta Medica, and Current Contents/Clinical Medicine (CC/CM).*

Contributors

CONSULTING EDITORS

RUSSELL R. LONSER, MD
Professor and Chair, Department of
Neurological Surgery, The Ohio State
University Wexner Medical Center, Columbus,
Ohio, USA

DANIEL K. RESNICK, MD, MS
Professor and Vice Chairman, Program
Director, Department of Neurosurgery,
University of Wisconsin-Madison School of
Medicine and Public Health, Madison,
Wisconsin, USA

EDITORS

JULIE G. PILITSIS, MD, PhD, MBA
Dean and Vice President of Medical Affairs,
Charles E. Schmidt College of Medicine,
Florida Atlantic University, Boca Raton, Florida,
USA

JOSHUA M. ROSENOW, MD
Professor of Neurosurgery, Neurology and
Physical Medicine and Rehabilitation,
Northwestern University Feinberg School of
Medicine, Department of Neurosurgery,
Chicago, Illinois, USA

AUTHORS

ELLEN L. AIR, MD, PhD
Department of Neurosurgery, Henry Ford
Hospital, Detroit, Michigan, USA

**ALEXANDER ALAMRI, MBBS, BSc, FHEA,
MRCS**
Neurosciences Research Centre, Molecular
and Clinical Sciences Institute, St George's
University of London, London, United Kingdom

RUSHNA ALI, MD
Department of Neurosciences, Spectrum
Health Medical Group, Michigan State
University, Grand Rapids, Michigan, USA

SAIM ALI, BA
Department of Neurological Surgery, New York
University Grossman School of Medicine, East
Meadow, NY, USA

JEFFREY E. ARLE, MD, PhD
Department of Neurosurgery, Beth Israel
Deaconess Medical Center, Department of
Neurosurgery, Harvard Medical School,
Boston, Massachusetts, USA; Department of

Neurosurgery, Mount Auburn Hospital,
Cambridge, Massachusetts, USA

JONATHAN BAO, BS
Department of Neuroscience and Experimental
Therapeutics, Albany Medical College, Albany,
New York, USA

AUSAF BARI, MD, PhD
Department of Neurosurgery, University of
California, Los Angeles, Los Angeles,
California, USA

BEN SHOFTY, MD, PhD
Department of Neurosurgery, Baylor College of
Medicine, Houston, Texas, USA

SHARONA BEN-HAIM, MD
Department of Neurosurgery, University of
California, San Diego, San Diego, California,
USA

MICHAEL G. BRANDEL, MD, MAS
Department of Neurosurgery, University of
California, San Diego, San Diego, California,
USA

JAMES CARUSO, MD
Department of Neurological Surgery, University of Texas Southwestern, Dallas, Texas, USA

HART P. FOGEL, BA
Columbia University Vagelos College of Physicians and Surgeons, New York, New York, USA

ELIZABETH E. GINALIS, MD
Department of Neurological Surgery, Rutgers-New Jersey Medical School, Newark, New Jersey, USA

AMIR HADANNY, MD
Department of Neurosurgery, Albany Medical College, Albany, New York, USA

TRAVIS M. HAMILTON, MD
Department of Neurosurgery, Henry Ford Hospital, Detroit, Michigan, USA

TESSA HARLAND, MD
Department of Neurosurgery, Albany Medical College, Albany, New York, USA

DEVON HENNEL, MS
Department of Neurscience & Experimental Therapeutics, Albany Medical College, Albany, NY, USA

ALON KASHANIAN, MD
Department of Surgery, Donald and Barbara Zucker School of Medicine at Hofstra/Northwell, Manhasset, New York, USA

ANTHONY KASPA ALLAM
Department of Neurosurgery, Baylor College of Medicine, Houston, Texas, USA

OLGA KHAZEN, MS
Department of Neurscience & Experimental Therapeutics, Albany Medical College, Albany, NY

CHRISTINE LIN, BA
Department of Neurosurgery, University of California, San Diego, San Diego, California, USA

DENNIS LONDON, MD
Department of Neurosurgery, Center for Neuromodulation, NYU Langone Health, New York, New York, USA

ANTONIOS MAMMIS, MD
Department of Neurological Surgery, New York University Grossman School of Medicine, East Meadow, NY, USA

M. BENJAMIN LARKIN, MD, PharmD
Department of Neurosurgery, Baylor College of Medicine, Houston, Texas, USA

ALON MOGILNER, MD, PhD
Department of Neurosurgery, Center for Neuromodulation, NYU Langone Health, New York, New York, USA

THIAGO S. MONTENEGRO, MD
Department of Neurosciences, Spectrum Health Medical Group, Michigan State University, Grand Rapids, Michigan, USA

ERLICK A.C. PEREIRA, MA(Camb), DM(Oxf), FRCS(NeuroSurg)
Neurosciences Research Centre, Molecular and Clinical Sciences Institute, St George's University of London, London, United Kingdom

JULIE G. PILITSIS, MD, PhD, MBA
Dean and Vice President of Medical Affairs, Charles E. Schmidt College of Medicine, Florida Atlantic University, Boca Raton, Florida, USA

NADER POURATIAN, MD, PhD
Department of Neurological Surgery, University of Texas Southwestern, Dallas, Texas, USA

JARED C. REESE, MD
Department of Neurosurgery, Henry Ford Hospital, Detroit, Michigan, USA

JOSHUA M. ROSENOW, MD
Professor of Neurosurgery, Neurology and Physical Medicine and Rehabilitation, Northwestern University Feinberg School of Medicine, Department of Neurosurgery, Chicago, Illinois, USA

JASON M. SCHWALB, MD, FAANS, FACS
Surgical Director, Movement Disorder and Comprehensive Epilepsy Centers, Henry Ford Medical Group, Research Scientist, Center for Health Policy and Health Services Research, Henry Ford Health, Clinical Professor, Wayne State University School of Medicine, West Bloomfield, Michigan, USA

NATHAN A. SHLOBIN, BA
Department of Neurological Surgery,
Northwestern University Feinberg School of
Medicine, Chicago, Illinois, USA

MICHAEL D. STAUDT, MD, MSc
Department of Neurosurgery, Oakland
University William Beaumont School of
Medicine, Rochester, Michigan, USA; Michigan
Head and Spine Institute, Southfield, Michigan,
USA; Assistant Professor, Department of
Neurosurgery Neuroscience Center, Beaumont
Health, Royal Oak, Michigan, USA

THOMAS TANGNEY, BS
Department of Neuroscience and Experimental
Therapeutics, Albany Medical College, Albany,
New York, USA

EVANGELIA TSOLAKI, PhD
Department of Neurosurgery, University of
California, Los Angeles, Los Angeles,
California, USA

ASHWIN VISWANATHAN, MD
Baylor College of Medicine, Houston, Texas,
USA

CHRISTOPHER J. WINFREE, MD, FAANS
Department of Neurological Surgery, Columbia
University, New York, New York,
USA

Contents

Preface: Advances in Pain Management   xiii

Julie G. Pilitsis and Joshua M. Rosenow

The Multidisciplinary Team in Pain Management   241

Michael D. Staudt

> A multidisciplinary approach to pain management includes evaluation by a variety of healthcare professionals who possess differing levels of expertise and who often consult with one another. The "core" multidisciplinary team commonly consists of primary care providers, anesthesiologists, psychologists, nurses, and physical and occupational therapists, with additional involvement from surgeons, neurologists, internists, physiatrists, psychiatrists, social workers, dietitians, and pharmacists. Multiple studies have supported the use of multidisciplinary programs as effective, cost-efficient, and superior to single-discipline treatments or outpatient nonmultidisciplinary rehabilitation; however, barriers to their implementation exist due to significant associated costs and need for longitudinal care.

Health Care Disparity in Pain   251

Travis M. Hamilton, Jared C. Reese, and Ellen L. Air

> Disparity in the treatment of chronic pain has become increasingly pertinent in health care, given the large burden of disease and its economic costs to society. That disease burden is disproportionally carried by minorities and those of lower socioeconomic status for a host of historical and systemic reasons. Only by understanding the cause of such disparities, collecting accurate and thorough data that illuminate all contributing factors, and diversifying the health care workforce, can we achieve more equitable treatment and reduce the burden of chronic pain.

Nonopioid Postoperative Pain Management in Neurosurgery   261

Nathan A. Shlobin and Joshua M. Rosenow

> Neurosurgeons have sought to minimize the use of opioids in neurosurgery. Preoperative medical strategies include methadone and gabapentinoids. Intraoperative strategies include local anesthetic infiltration with bupivacaine, ropivacaine, and lidocaine; scalp block; steroids such as methylprednisolone, triamcinolone, and dexamethasone; ketamine; acetaminophen; ketorolac; liposomal bupivacaine; dexmedetomidine; and performing awake surgery. Postoperative strategies include continuous infusion pumps, wound catheters, and patient-controlled analgesia. Multimodal analgesia may be most effective, with the enhanced recovery after surgery (ERAS) pathway as an example and cognitive-behavioral therapy (CBT) as an adjunct. Patient-specific demographics and clinical factors must be considered in selecting the appropriate approach for a given patient.

Mindfulness Meditation in the Treatment of Chronic Pain   275

Michael G. Brandel, Christine Lin, Devon Hennel, Olga Khazen, Julie G. Pilitsis, and Sharona Ben-Haim

> Chronic pain is a leading cause of disability in the United States. Limited efficacy associated with pharmacologic management and surgical interventions in refractory patients has led to further exploration of cognitive and behavioral interventions as both an adjunctive and primary therapeutic modality. Mindfulness-based meditation has shown to be effective in reducing pain in randomized studies of chronic pain patients as well as models of experimentally induced pain in healthy participants. These studies have revealed specific neural mechanisms which may explain both short-term and sustained pain relief associated with mindfulness-based interventions.

Financial Sustainability of Neuromodulation for Pain   281

Jason M. Schwalb

> When considering the financial sustainability of neuromodulation for pain, one needs to consider the varying costs involved with this therapy. These include comparisons between different types of neuromodulation, comparisons between neuromodulation and conventional therapy, and comparisons between neuromodulation and other invasive modalities. In addition, any consideration of cost also needs to take quality into account. Even if a therapy is expensive, it can be considered cost-effective if it leads to significant increase in quality of life and economic productivity of the patient. This review considers these questions, methodologies used to assess them, and variations between different health delivery systems.

Spinal Cord Stimulation: New Waveforms and Technology   287

Dennis London and Alon Mogilner

> The efficacy of spinal cord stimulation for treating chronic pain has encouraged the development of a wide variety of different technologies for stimulation. In this review, the authors first discuss how parameters of stimulation determine the stimulation waveform. They then discuss new stimulation waveforms, including high frequency and burst stimulation, and the evidence supporting their use. Finally, the authors turn to emerging technologies and techniques including dorsal root ganglion stimulation, wireless stimulation, and closed-loop stimulation.

Closed-Loop Systems in Neuromodulation: Electrophysiology and Wearables   297

Thiago S. Montenegro, Rushna Ali, and Jeffrey E. Arle

> Most currently available neuromodulation techniques for pain work through an open-loop system. The distance between the epidural space and the target of the stimulation in a dynamic body can change because of physiologic conditions. The closed-loop system in spinal cord neuromodulation consists of an integrated system that records real-time electrophysiological activity in the form of evoked compound action potentials and uses it in a feedback mechanism to adjust stimulus output. Wearables represent newly developed technologies that have gained traction in recent years. Their application in pain management is still developing but promising.

The Role of Intrathecal Pumps in Nonmalignant Pain   305

Elizabeth E. Ginalis, Saim Ali, and Antonios Mammis

Intrathecal pumps deliver analgesic medication directly into the central nervous system. In patients with chronic nonmalignant pain, intrathecal therapy using morphine or ziconotide has been shown to be an effective option when traditional noninvasive methods do not provide adequate relief. There has been increasing use of intrathecal drug administration in the management of patients with nonmalignant pain in recent years given the advances in technology and research on the topic. However, due to its invasive nature, intrathecal pumps remain the last option among patients with chronic pain.

Deep Brain Stimulation for Chronic Pain   311

Alexander Alamri and Erlick A.C. Pereira

Deep brain stimulation (DBS) is a neurosurgical intervention well known for the treatment of movement disorders as well as epilepsy, Tourette syndrome, and obsessive-compulsive disorders. DBS was pioneered in the 1950s, however, as a tool for treating facial pain, phantom limb pain, post-stroke pain, and brachial plexus pain among other disease states. Various anatomic targets exist, including the sensory thalamus (ventral posterior lateral and ventral posterior medial), the periaqueductal gray and periventricular gray matter, and the anterior cingulate cortex.

What's New in Peripheral Nerve Stimulation   323

Hart P. Fogel and Christopher J. Winfree

Peripheral nerve stimulation (PNS) is a powerful interventional option for the management of otherwise intractable pain. This technique involves the implantation of electrodes to apply electrical stimulation to named peripheral nerves, thereby alleviating pain in the territory of the target nerves. Recent advancements, largely driven by physician-industry relationships, have transformed the therapy into one that is minimally-invasive, safe, evidence-based, and effective. Ongoing research has expanded the indications beyond chronic neuropathic pain in a peripheral nerve distribution. This article provides an overview of recent advances in this field.

Focused Ultrasound for Chronic Pain   331

Jonathan Bao, Thomas Tangney, and Julie G. Pilitsis

Chronic pain affects millions of Americans and is one of the leading reasons for individuals to seek medical attention. Focused ultrasound has been studied as a noninvasive treatment option for various pain disorders. Current studies have used focused ultrasound for ablation, neuromodulation, and opening of the blood-brain barrier for drug and therapy delivery. Most of the work has been performed in ablative studies and has shown efficacy in treating chronic neuropathic pain. Further research is needed to expand its usage in neurosurgery.

Ablation Procedures   339

Anthony Kaspa Allam, M. Benjamin Larkin, Ben Shofty, and Ashwin Viswanathan

Although ablation has a limited role in the management of chronic noncancer pain, ablation continues to help patients with treatment of refractory cancer-related pain. Interdisciplinary treatment involving supportive care, pain medicine, oncology, and

neurosurgery is critical to optimizing the timing and outcome of neurosurgical ablative options for pain management. In this review, 3 targets for ablative surgery—the
spinothalamic tract, the dorsal column's visceral pain pathway, and the anterior
cingulate cortex—are discussed with a focus on patient selection and key aspects
of surgical technique.

Imaging as a Pain Biomarker   345

Alon Kashanian, Evangelia Tsolaki, James Caruso, Ausaf Bari, and Nader Pouratian

In recent years, the hunt for objective biomarkers in chronic pain has intensified, as
interest has grown in precision medicine techniques, and the global opioid crisis has
underscored the need to accelerate the pace of pain research. A growing body of
neuroimaging literature suggests that chronic pain is associated with various alterations in regional brain areas as well as whole-brain networks, which may represent
unique radiological pain signatures or biomarkers to guide diagnosis, response, and
treatment. Here, we provide a comprehensive and updated literature review on
investigative efforts to identify neuroimaging biomarkers for pain.

Machine Learning and Pain Outcomes   351

Tessa Harland, Amir Hadanny, and Julie G. Pilitsis

Machine learning (ML) is an increasingly popular method of data analysis that has
meaningful application within the realm of pain management. Current research
has used this technique as a tool to refine patient selection for more invasive pain
management treatments in an effort to improve outcomes. It is also being used to
aid in the search for biomarkers that could objectify the quantification of pain to better assess these outcomes. This article provides an overview of ML and its applications within the pain field.

NEUROSURGERY CLINICS OF NORTH AMERICA

FORTHCOMING ISSUES

October 2022
Update on Open Vascular Surgery
Michael T. Lawton, *Editor*

January 2023
Chiari I Malformation
David D. Limbrick and Jeffrey Leonard, *Editors*

RECENT ISSUES

April 2022
Recent Advances in Endovascular Neurosurgery
Elad I. Levy, Azam S. Ahmed, and Justin M. Cappuzzo, *Editors*

January 2022
Syndromic Neurosurgery
James A. Stadler III and Mari L. Groves, *Editors*

SERIES OF RELATED INTEREST

Neurologic Clinics
https://www.neurologic.theclinics.com/
Neuroimaging Clinics
https://www.neuroimaging.theclinics.com/

THE CLINICS ARE AVAILABLE ONLINE!
Access your subscription at:
www.theclinics.com

Preface
Advances in Pain Management

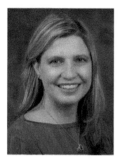 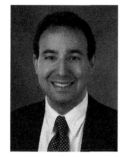

Julie G. Pilitsis, MD, PhD, MBA   Joshua M. Rosenow, MD

Editors

Recent events have highlighted the need for better management of chronic pain. Pain is one of the most common reasons for an individual to visit the emergency room and one of the most common reasons for surgery. Neurosurgeons are often performing procedures for the purposes of managing pain, whether that be radiculopathy, trigeminal neuralgia, chronic regional pain syndrome, or peripheral nerve entrapment. This issue of *Neurosurgery Clinics of North America* explores multiple diverse aspects of neurosurgical pain care. Some of the articles herein describe the composition and organization of a multidisciplinary pain team as well as the socioeconomic aspects of running a neurosurgical pain program. The content also touches on methods of treating postoperative pain while minimizing the use of opioids. Several of the articles describe some of the advances that have moved older modalities, such as spinal cord stimulation and intrathecal medication delivery, into the twenty-first century. Moreover, other existing procedures, such as ablative therapies and deep brain stimulation, also get a fresh viewpoint given the current state of devices and knowledge. In addition, there are contributions touching on some of the strides being made in identifying imaging biomarkers to aid in tracking outcomes from pain treatment. Last, this collection explores emerging trends in focused ultrasound and machine learning. We hope that this content proves useful to the practicing neurosurgeon and stimulating to those who are considering concentrating their work in this evolving specialty.

Julie G. Pilitsis, MD, PhD, MBA
Charles E. Schmidt College of Medicine, Florida
Atlantic University, 777 Glades Road BC-71, Boca
Raton, FL 33431, USA

Joshua M. Rosenow, MD
Department of Neurosurgery
Northwestern University
Feinberg School of Medicine
676 North St Clair Street, Suite 2210
Chicago, IL 60611, USA

E-mail addresses:
jpilitsis@health.fau.edu (J.G. Pilitsis)
jrosenow@nm.org (J.M. Rosenow)

Neurosurg Clin N Am 33 (2022) xiii
https://doi.org/10.1016/j.nec.2022.03.002
1042-3680/22/© 2022 Published by Elsevier Inc.

The Multidisciplinary Team in Pain Management

Michael D. Staudt, MD, MSc[a,b,c,*]

KEYWORDS

- Biopsychosocial • Chronic pain • Collaboration • Interdisciplinary • Multidisciplinary
- Neuromodulation • Neurosurgery • Pain management

KEY POINTS

- The composition of multidisciplinary pain teams is variable and can include primary care providers, anesthesiologists, psychologists, nurses, physical and occupational therapists, surgeons, neurologists, physiatrists, psychiatrists, social workers, dietitians, and pharmacists.
- Although assembling a multidisciplinary team is important, it is essential to foster open communication between team members and patients.
- Multidisciplinary programs are clinically effective, cost-efficient, and superior to single-discipline treatments or outpatient non-multidisciplinary rehabilitation for the treatment of chronic pain.
- Neurosurgeons are leaders in the study of chronic pain and implementation of evidence-based guidelines and have an important role on multidisciplinary pain teams.

INTRODUCTION

Pain-related complaints are the primary reason for patients to seek medical care or visit an emergency department in the United States.[1] Pain afflicts patients acutely and chronically, and it is important to recognize the distinct treatment approaches applicable to both of these pathologies. In particular, the management of chronic pain demands attention to biological, psychological and social factors–such a biopsychosocial approach is an important consideration that influences the perception and coping of pain.[2] Accordingly, the management of chronic pain is complex, and often requires the expertise and resources of multiple disciplines. As such, a multidisciplinary approach is preferred to optimize all facets of chronic pain management, delivering a high level of individualized care.

A multidisciplinary approach to pain management includes evaluation by a variety of healthcare professionals who possess differing levels of expertise and who often consult with one another. Coordinated treatment may involve medications, surgery, physical therapy, and/or cognitive-behavioral therapy. There is no specific composition of a multidisciplinary team, although the "core" players tend to include primary care physicians, pain physicians, nurses, physical therapists, and psychologists. Depending on the etiology of pain, this core group can be expanded to include surgeons, psychiatrists, and physiatrists, although there is no "one size fits all" mentality.

It is important to recognize that patients with chronic pain require longitudinal care with frequent provider visits and re-evaluation of both therapies and goals of care, which can lead to the multidisciplinary team members changing dynamically over time. Equally important is to recognize that some patients are "seeking a cure that does not exist,"[3] which can cause distress and dissatisfaction among patients and providers, and should prompt a continuous re-evaluation of expectations and treatment goals. An individualized approach is

[a] Department of Neurosurgery, Neuroscience Center, Beaumont Health, Royal Oak, MI, USA; [b] Department of Neurosurgery, Oakland University William Beaumont School of Medicine, Rochester, MI, USA; [c] Michigan Head and Spine Institute, Southfield, MI, USA

* Department of Neurosurgery, Neuroscience Center, Beaumont Health, 3555 13 Mile Road, N220, Royal Oak, MI 48073.

E-mail address: Michael.Staudt@beaumont.org

Neurosurg Clin N Am 33 (2022) 241–249
https://doi.org/10.1016/j.nec.2022.02.002

1042-3680/22/© 2022 Elsevier Inc. All rights reserved.

essential, as patients will perceive treatment as insufficient if it does not align with their specific needs.[4]

Although multidisciplinary pain programs have been defined in various ways,[5] the International Association for the Study of Pain has created a set of guidelines that distinguish between multidisciplinary pain centers and multidisciplinary pain clinics.[6] Multidisciplinary pain centers are considered part of or are affiliated with a higher education institution or research center. These centers coordinate care with providers from different specialties within the same space, with an emphasis placed on comprehensive care that adheres to treatment guidelines, strives for continuous quality improvement, and actively engages in research pursuits. In comparison, a multidisciplinary pain clinic strives to offer the same level of care and expertise, although are not necessarily associated with an active academic or research mandate.

Regardless of definition, multidisciplinary programs have demonstrated clinical efficacy as well as cost-efficiency.[7] The goal of this article is to review the multidisciplinary management of chronic pain through a historical and contemporary perspective, with a focus on the multidisciplinary team members and the role of the neurosurgeon.

A HISTORICAL PERSPECTIVE
The Origins of Pain Medicine as a Multidisciplinary Field

One of the earliest proponents of the multidisciplinary team approach chronic pain was Dr. John Bonica, an anesthesiologist. During World War II, he was assigned to treat military personnel with various pain problems—he became acutely aware that patients with chronic pain conditions responded inadequately to treatment compared to patients with more straightforward pain problems, and also that there was a lack of research, literature, and training on managing patients with chronic pain.[8] He thereafter sought consultation from colleagues in other disciplines and soon realized that independent consultations were inefficient and delayed optimal care.[8] Following the war, he went on to develop one of the first multidisciplinary programs in Tacoma, Washington, which consisted of an anesthesiologist, neurosurgeon, orthopedic surgeon, psychiatrist, and radiation therapist.

Following the establishment of multidisciplinary programs in the 1950s, there was slow initial growth over the next 2 decades. Then, interest in pain research and management surged in the late 1960s and early 1970s thanks to the

publication of the gate control theory of pain and the establishment of the International Association for the Study of Pain.[8,9] Accordingly, the number of pain treatment facilities grew rapidly in the United States, numbering over 1000 by 1990.[10]

Multiple studies and systematic reviews have supported the use of multidisciplinary programs as effective, cost-efficient, and superior to single-discipline treatments or outpatient non-multidisciplinary rehabilitation. Such positive outcomes include improvements in pain severity and mood, and also reduced opioid use, improved function, and increased rates of returning to work.[11–14] Furthermore, gains as a result of multidisciplinary treatment have reportedly been maintained well beyond the initial treatment period.[15]

Unfortunately, despite a robust body of clinical evidence, multidisciplinary programs in the United States saw a decline in the 2000s, which has been attributed to the influence of the insurance industry and hospital administration, although the true reason is multifactorial.[16,17] Certainly, the upfront cost of an intensive treatment program is steep, which is anathema to third-party payers; however, the evidence supporting the long-term cost-effectiveness should provide a compelling counter-argument.[14,16] Moreover, the ease of prescribing pharmaceutical treatments such as opioids, combined with the incentivization of interventional procedures saw a shift in prioritization and reimbursement. In fact, many third-party payers tend to "carve out" services to save costs, defeating the purpose of a multidisciplinary program. Robbins and colleagues[18] described this as "disconnected" health care professionals without coordination, which has a negative impact on chronic pain relief.

Pain and the Opioid Crisis

It would be remiss not to mention the ongoing opioid crisis, and how it relates to a multidisciplinary approach to pain. From the mid-1990s to the early 2000s, key national institutions including the Department of Veterans Affairs and the Joint Commission recognized pain as the "Fifth Vital Sign"[19]; however, its implementation did little to improve pain outcomes in any clinical setting.[20] Furthermore, attempting to treat the "numerical" value of pain has exacerbated the opioid crisis, leading the American Medical Association recommending the "Fifth Vital Sign" to be removed in 2016.[20]

The "Fifth Vital Sign" campaign saw increased use of opioids to treat pain, which arguably led to changing the dynamic of physician and patient expectations for what pain management entailed.

An unintended consequence of focusing on patient-centered care and satisfaction surveys saw a paradoxic increase in opioid prescribing.[21,22] This also gave rise to so-called "pill mill" clinics, which have been advertised as multidisciplinary pain clinics, but did little more than push opioid prescriptions.[17]

There were 76 million prescriptions for opioids in 1991, compared to 219 million prescriptions in 2011.[23] As a result, the rise in opioid prescriptions has fostered misuse, abuse and addiction. In 2016, 11.5 million people in the U.S. were abusing opioids and 2.1 million had developed opioid use disorder.[23] Prescription opioids are freely shared among families and friends–more than 50% of users stated that they obtained opioids from a friend or a relative for free.[24] Unfortunately, even in cases where medications are taken as prescribed, addiction can occur, leading to the risk of subsequent abuse and overdose. Unsurprisingly, a third of overdose-related deaths are linked with pharmaceutical opioids as opposed to only 19% associated with heroin.[25] Additionally, opioid-related overdose deaths have grown rapidly over the past 2 decades, from less than 10,000 in 1999 to greater than 40,000 in 2016.[23] Currently, opioids continue to be the most-often prescribed pain medication class in the United States.[25]

The treatment of chronic pain requires careful attention to medication management, including selecting appropriate medications and dosages, and managing tolerance and side effects. Accordingly, many primary care providers lack the training, experience, and comfort of dealing with chronic pain management and opioid use disorder.[26] Some studies have reported the integration of a clinical pharmacist into a multidisciplinary setting, with improved adherence to screening and practice standards, and a reduction in morphine equivalent dose values.[27,28] Ultimately, active medication management is necessary to reduce opioid doses, which requires a concerted effort by a multidisciplinary team and often changing the primary opioid prescriber.[29]

The Current State of Multidisciplinary Facilities

Multidisciplinary treatment facilities for chronic pain are considered the highest standard of care; however, there is a distinct lack of research and reporting on the prevalence and composition of such programs. As expected, there is considerable variability in the availability and services provided by multidisciplinary pain clinics within the United States and other countries, including Australia, Canada, and the United Kingdom.[30]

One of the key points is that there is a mismatch between supply and demand, with few treatment facilities available but high caseload volume and long wait times.[30,31] A common theme is a need for improved access to multidisciplinary pain teams and facilities.

As mentioned, there are a number of factors that impede access to multidisciplinary pain programs, particularly in the United States. Meldrum and colleagues[32] succinctly identified three core issues: (1) most centers often segment medical professionals by discipline as opposed to encouraging collaboration; (2) fee-for-service models favor procedures, such as spinal injections and spine surgeries, over time-intensive assessments and behavioral therapy; and (3) multidisciplinary programs require individualized treatment and behavioral change, compared to the relative "ease" of a surgical or medical intervention. Ultimately, this third point may be driven by the patients themselves.[32,33]

THE MULTIDISCIPLINARY TEAM
Team Composition and Key Players

Multidisciplinary teams can be structured differently depending on the region in which they operate, and also based on the needs of the local patient population. Furthermore, the structure and composition of the team depend on the medical setting, including academic versus community-based hospitals, group practices, and walk-in clinics, for example. Accordingly, what is considered the "core" of the multidisciplinary team can vary, although commonly there is involvement from primary care providers, anesthesiologists, psychologists, nurses, and physical and occupational therapists.[34] Additional specialists can include surgeons, neurologists, internists, physiatrists, psychiatrists, social workers, dietitians, and pharmacists.

It is important to recognize that there is no dedicated residency training program for pain management. In the United States, board certification is available through a 1-year fellowship program accredited by the Accreditation Council for Graduate Medical Education. Candidacy first requires the completion of residency in primary care, anesthesiology, neurology, or physical medicine and rehabilitation, for example, which also likely influences how each provider approaches a particular patient or pain syndrome. Furthermore, different states have different requirements regarding policies that govern pain management clinics, or even the definition of what a "pain specialist" is.[35]

Whereas multidisciplinary treatment is defined by having three or more health care providers from different disciplines, integration and collaboration is perhaps the most important facet. It has been reported that, even in a multidisciplinary setting, not all team members may truly be integrated due to the lack of communication and lack of regular meetings to discuss patient care.[34,36] As such, effective care is more than assembling the key players; it is also creating an interdisciplinary approach.[34]

Roles and Responsibilities

The first point of contact is often within primary care, and it is often challenging for front-line providers to diagnose and manage complex pain presentations and addiction[37]; however, these providers play an instrumental role in the first assessment leading to a potential diagnosis, managing medications, and treating comorbidities including anxiety and depression. Primary care physicians are often considered the gatekeeper–depending on the nature and complexity of the pain diagnosis, the most important first step is often identifying the problem and providing the appropriate referral to other healthcare providers. Another important facet of initial care is in the emergency department; however, chronic pain patients often demonstrate complex needs which are difficult to address in an acute care environment.[38]

Primary care providers often find themselves dealing with balancing the treatment of chronic pain with the development of opioid use disorders. Accordingly, surveys of primary care providers report an overall low satisfaction and confidence in treating chronic pain, which can lead to provider burnout and patient dissatisfaction.[39] For some providers, offering a multidisciplinary consultation service to review cases and provide advice and management recommendations may offer an avenue for increased support and confidence in treatment.[37] Furthermore, it has been suggested that overcoming barriers to chronic pain care can be mitigated by improving education and competency in chronic pain management among primary care providers.[17]

It should be emphasized that many chronic pain conditions can be treated within primary care, although refractory pain and more challenging pain presentations such as complex regional pain syndrome necessitate an earlier assessment by specialists. Ultimately, the decision to refer to a specialist is multifactorial, and improved provider education and support will foster more appropriate and timely referrals of chronic pain patients who require a more specialized treatment approach.

Anesthesiologists are a common component of the core team and are dually trained in the administration of analgesic drugs and the use of interventional procedures. Such interventional procedures include nerve blocks, radiofrequency ablations, or the implantation of neuromodulation devices. Procedures can also be performed by other subspecialists including physiatrists and neurologists. Physiatrists are also able to emphasize rehabilitation techniques to improve mobility and function, whereas neurologists are able to provide a comprehensive neurologic assessment that can help localize an anatomic or neurologic source of pain.

Mental health is equally as important as alleviating the physical painful stimulus, if not more so. Many multidisciplinary teams include a psychologist to help manage the psychosocial aspect of pain management, and these providers can help identify poor coping strategies in patients and initiate cognitive-behavioral therapies to remove learned behaviors and manage negative associations. Chronic pain is also confounded by mental health disorders, such as depression, anxiety, and post-traumatic stress disorders. As such, psychiatrists also have an important role to play in helping to recognize and diagnose underlying pathologies and recommending the appropriate pharmacologic management. The management of psychiatric comorbidities has important implications for management–one study of chronic pain patients undergoing spinal cord stimulation reported that those patients with comorbid depression, anxiety, substance abuse, or a history of abuse were more likely to undergo removal of their device within 1 year, primarily due to lack of efficacy.[40] Depression has also been linked with poorer outcomes and satisfaction following spine surgery.[41,42]

Nurses and allied healthcare professionals are often the cornerstone for the implementation of pain management strategies and providing day-to-day care. Nurses have a frontline role and often have the most contact with patients; accordingly, they are able to provide ongoing assessment regarding the efficacy of pain management strategies, in addition to encouraging treatment adherence and dispensing medication advice.[43] Physical therapists are essential in designing and implementing treatment plans that can include therapeutic stretching, exercise, and massage. In fact, physical therapists have been reported to receive more hours of pain-relevant training than medical students, highlighting the importance of their knowledge and experience.[43,44]

The Role of the Neurosurgeon

Neurosurgeons have played an important role in the treatment of chronic pain since the inception of the specialty, particularly for pain conditions such as trigeminal neuralgia and degenerative spine disease. As the field has evolved, medical technologies have become increasingly sophisticated and prevalent in the treatment of chronic pain, and neuromodulation modalities have emerged as an essential component of a multidisciplinary approach to pain management. Common pain conditions treated with neuromodulation include post-laminectomy syndrome, complex regional pain syndrome, craniofacial pain syndromes, central pain syndromes including post-stroke pain, and peripheral pain syndromes including diabetic neuropathy, among others.

Innovation in medical technologies has rapidly expanded the indications for treatment; as such, the role of the neurosurgeon has evolved and expanded. This has also led to significant treatment overlap with other physicians–for example, spinal cord stimulators, peripheral nerve stimulators, and intrathecal pumps can be implanted by neurosurgeons or interventional pain practitioners. Due to the breadth and complexity of pain conditions, and the variety of treatment options available, this has expanded the dialogue between specialties and fostered communication and collaboration.

Neurosurgeons are leaders in the study of chronic pain and implementation of evidence-based guidelines, as demonstrated by high-quality publications on the treatment of post-laminectomy syndrome,[45,46] complex regional pain syndrome,[47] occipital neuralgia,[48] and diabetic neuropathy.[49] Importantly, these publications are coauthored by a diverse group of clinicians and researchers from different specialties, highlighting the importance of a multidisciplinary approach in advancing the study and treatment of chronic pain.

There are various multidisciplinary efforts for the treatment of complex pain syndromes for which neurosurgeons are actively involved, often taking a primary role. Two relevant examples are Enhanced Recovery After Surgery (ERAS) protocols and pelvic pain consortiums.

Enhanced Recovery After Surgery

Inadequate postoperative pain control is associated with harmful physiologic side effects, poor patient satisfaction, and an increased overall cost of healthcare resource utilization.[50] As such, the philosophy of ERAS consists of a multimodal approach to perioperative management and optimization, with the implementation of evidence-based approaches to treatment.[51] The development of ERAS protocols were also spurred by the abundant use of opioids for the treatment of acute postoperative pain, thus giving rise to multimodal analgesic paradigms to reduce opioid use

and improve postoperative pain control and patient recovery.[52,53] Within neurosurgery, ERAS has been applied most commonly in spinal surgery,[54,55] and neurosurgeons have been some of the most important innovators in the field.[56]

ERAS protocols require a multidisciplinary, team-based approach, and typically institutions have developed their own protocols to address the needs of their patients. The development of an ERAS protocol requires the coordination of team-based meetings and open communication with patients, allied healthcare professional, physicians, and other ancillary healthcare providers. The first consideration is the preoperative optimization of medical comorbidities with the involvement of primary care providers, nurse practitioners, and physical therapists. Intraoperatively, the anesthesia team and operating room staff are critical for implementing the appropriate strategies. Postoperative care then employs pain management algorithms and early mobilization; this often requires the expertise and involvement of residents, mid-level providers, and hospitalists.

Most published ERAS studies have described an overall benefit, including reduced opioid usage, decreased length of stay, and a reduction in complications and readmissions[57]; however, their implementation is lacking.[58] The focus on a multidisciplinary approach encompassing the preoperative to the postoperative phase is appealing and deserves more attention and promotion.

Pelvic Pain

Chronic pelvic pain is a debilitating, multifactorial condition with the involvement of gynecologic, urologic, gastrointestinal, musculoskeletal, and psychiatric components. Pelvic pain is often misunderstood and misdiagnosed, and multiple specialties are often involved due to the complexity of diagnosis and management. In particular, pelvic pain patients present a therapeutic challenge as their duration of pain is often long prior to diagnosis and treatment.[59] Diagnosis is typically delayed by as much as 10 years, and resulting in significant emotional and physiologic challenges.[59]

A multidisciplinary approach is essential, as each specialty provides a certain level of expertise. Such an approach has been reported to address organic and psychological aspects of pain to promote a more thorough and efficacious treatment plan, compared to single-discipline treatments.[60] The core team often includes a gynecologist, anesthesiologist, urologist, gastroenterologist, psychologist, and physiotherapist.

A variety of treatment paradigms have been employed including physical therapy, medications, pudendal nerve blocks, and botulinum toxin injection; however, treatment success is limited and pain often refractory.[61] Accordingly, neurosurgeons have an increasing role in the management of pelvic pain with neuromodulation therapies such as spinal cord stimulation, dorsal root ganglion stimulation, and intrathecal pain pumps.[62] A comprehensive workflow for the diagnosis and management of pelvic pain, including the successful identification of candidates for neuromodulation, has recently been described, which can provide the framework for establishing a multidisciplinary pelvic pain consortium.[63]

ENSURING SUCCESS

Optimizing the treatment of chronic pain requires a collaborative approach to patient care, including the judicious use of medications, psychological counseling, physical therapy, and surgical or interventional procedures. Equally important is ensuring open communication between multidisciplinary team members and patients.[64] Communication breakdown can occur between providers, such as with incomplete or inadequate referrals that do not provide a complete clinical picture, or between the provider and patient. For example, it is common for patients to think that their symptoms are not taken seriously.[65] The adverse effects of poor communication can lead to improper management, inadequate pain relief, and missed diagnoses. Furthermore, barriers exist that contribute to the lack of access to chronic pain management, including socioeconomic and racial disparities, lack of financial means to accessing specialty care, and the deficiency of specialized programs in rural areas.[17,66]

Also important is managing patient expectations—for example, some patients undergoing spinal cord stimulation for post-laminectomy syndrome may have unrealistic expectations of pain relief, sleep and return to work.[67] The goal of neuromodulation, and of all pain therapies, is not to eliminate pain but to improve quality of life. Patients must take an active role in their care, such as enacting lifestyle changes and actively participating in medication reduction and physical therapy. Ultimately, patient education within a multidisciplinary chronic pain program is important to improve both the treatment efficacy and patient self-management.[68]

SUMMARY

Medicine in the modern era is built on collaboration. Accordingly, a multidisciplinary approach to chronic pain management is essential due to its complexity. Although the composition of such teams can vary, it is important that they function in an integrated manner to promote interdisciplinary collaboration. There also remains significant variability in the implementation and standardization of multidisciplinary pain programs; however, the clinical efficacy and cost-effectiveness afforded by such programs have been well-established. As such, it is essential to continue to foster collaboration in chronic pain management and develop educational and organizational standards, which will ultimately help advance clinical excellence and patient care.

CLINICS CARE POINTS

- Patients with chronic pain require longitudinal care with frequent provider visits and re-evaluation of both therapies and goals of care, which can lead to the multidisciplinary team members changing dynamically over time.

- Effective multidisciplinary care is more than assembling the key players – it also requires an interdisciplinary approach.

- Mental health is equally as important as alleviating the physical painful stimulus, if not more so.

- The goal of pain management is not to eliminate pain entirely, but to improve quality of life; thus managing patient expectations is essential.

DISCLOSURE

The author reports no conflict of interest concerning the materials or methods used in this study or the findings specified in this article.

REFERENCES

1. Chang HY, Daubresse M, Kruszewski SP, et al. Prevalence and treatment of pain in EDs in the United States, 2000 to 2010. Am J Emerg Med 2014; 32(5):421–31.
2. Gatchel RJ, Peng YB, Peters ML, et al. The biopsychosocial approach to chronic pain: scientific advances and future directions. Psychol Bull 2007; 133(4):581–624.
3. Clare A, MacNeil S, Bunton T, et al. The Doctor doesn't need to see you now': reduction in general practice appointments following group pain management. Br J Pain 2019;13(2):121–9.

4. Nost TH, Steinsbekk A. A lifebuoy' and 'a waste of time': patients' varying experiences of multidisciplinary pain centre treatment- a qualitative study. BMC Health Serv Res 2019;19(1):1015.

5. Kaiser U, Arnold B, Pfingsten M, et al. Multidisciplinary pain management programs. J Pain Res 2013;6:355–8.

6. International Association for the Study of Pain. Pain treatment services. 2021. Available at: https://www.iasp-pain.org/resources/guidelines/pain-treatment-services/. Accessed September 26, 2021.

7. Turk DC. Clinical effectiveness and cost-effectiveness of treatments for patients with chronic pain. Clin J pain 2002;18(6):355–65.

8. Bonica JJ. Evolution and current status of pain programs. J Pain Symptom Manage 1990;5(6):368–74.

9. Melzack R, Wall PD. Pain mechanisms: a new theory. Science 1965;150(3699):971–9.

10. Okifuji A, Turk DC. Philosophy and efficacy of multidisciplinary approach to chronic pain management. J Anesth 1998;12(3):142–52.

11. Flor H, Fydrich T, Turk DC. Efficacy of multidisciplinary pain treatment centers: a meta-analytic review. Pain 1992;49(2):221–30.

12. Guzman J, Esmail R, Karjalainen K, et al. Multidisciplinary rehabilitation for chronic low back pain: systematic review. BMJ 2001;322(7301):1511–6.

13. Kamper SJ, Apeldoorn AT, Chiarotto A, et al. Multidisciplinary biopsychosocial rehabilitation for chronic low back pain: Cochrane systematic review and meta-analysis. BMJ 2015;350:h444.

14. Clark TS. Interdisciplinary treatment for chronic pain: is it worth the money? Proc (Bayl Univ Med Cent) 2000;13(3):240–3.

15. Patrick LE, Altmaier EM, Found EM. Long-term outcomes in multidisciplinary treatment of chronic low back pain: results of a 13-year follow-up. Spine 2004;29(8):850–5.

16. Schatman ME. The demise of multidisciplinary pain management clinics?. 2011. Available at: https://www.practicalpainmanagement.com/resources/practice-management/demise-multidisciplinary-pain-management-clinics. Accessed October 9, 2021.

17. Gatchel RJ, McGeary DD, McGeary CA, et al. Interdisciplinary chronic pain management: past, present, and future. Am Psychol 2014;69(2):119–30.

18. Robbins H, Gatchel RJ, Noe C, et al. A prospective one-year outcome study of interdisciplinary chronic pain management: compromising its efficacy by managed care policies. Anesth Analg 2003;97(1):156–62. table of contents.

19. Department of Veterans Affairs. Pain: The Fifth Vital Sign 2000. Available at: https://www.va.gov/painmanagement/docs/pain_as_the_5th_vital_sign_toolkit.pdf.

20. Scher C, Meador L, Van Cleave JH, et al. Moving beyond pain as the fifth vital sign and patient satisfaction scores to improve pain care in the 21st century. Pain Manag Nurs 2018;19(2):125–9.

21. Tompkins DA, Hobelmann JG, Compton P. Providing chronic pain management in the "Fifth Vital Sign" Era: Historical and treatment perspectives on a modern-day medical dilemma. Drug Alcohol Depend 2017;173(Suppl 1):S11–21.

22. Zgierska A, Miller M, Rabago D. Patient satisfaction, prescription drug abuse, and potential unintended consequences. JAMA 2012;307(13):1377–8.

23. Hagemeier NE. Introduction to the opioid epidemic: the economic burden on the healthcare system and impact on quality of life. Am J Manag Care 2018;24(10 Suppl):S200–6.

24. Jones CM, Paulozzi LJ, Mack KA. Sources of prescription opioid pain relievers by frequency of past-year nonmedical use United States, 2008-2011. JAMA Intern Med 2014;174(5):802–3.

25. Volkow ND, McLellan AT. Opioid abuse in chronic pain–misconceptions and mitigation strategies. N Engl J Med 2016;374(13):1253–63.

26. Harder VS, Villanti AC, Heil SH, et al. Opioid use disorder treatment in rural settings: the primary care perspective. Prev Med 2021;106765.

27. Boren LL, Locke AM, Friedman AS, et al. Team-based medicine: incorporating a clinical pharmacist into pain and opioid practice management. PM R 2019;11(11):1170–7.

28. Slipp M, Burnham R. Medication management of chronic pain: A comparison of 2 care delivery models. Can Pharm J 2017;150(2):112–7.

29. Sud A, Armas A, Cunningham H, et al. Multidisciplinary care for opioid dose reduction in patients with chronic non-cancer pain: a systematic realist review. PloS one 2020;15(7):e0236419.

30. Fashler SR, Cooper LK, Oosenbrug ED, et al. Systematic review of multidisciplinary chronic pain treatment facilities. Pain Res Manag 2016;2016:5960987.

31. Deslauriers S, Roy JS, Bernatsky S, et al. The burden of waiting to access pain clinic services: perceptions and experiences of patients with rheumatic conditions. BMC Health Serv Res 2021;21(1):160.

32. Meldrum ML. Brief history of multidisciplinary management of chronic pain, 1900-2000. In: Schatman ME, Campbell A, editors. Chronic pain management: guidelines for multidisciplinary program development. New York: Informa Healthcare USA; 2007. p. 1–13.

33. Jeffery MM, Butler M, Stark A, et al. In: Multidisciplinary pain programs for chronic noncancer pain. Rockville (MD). Agency for Healthcare Research and Quality (US; 2011.

34. Peng P, Stinson JN, Choiniere M, et al. Role of health care professionals in multidisciplinary pain treatment facilities in Canada. Pain Res Manag 2008;13(6):484–8.

35. Bennett K. Can i call myself a "pain specialist?". 2019. Available at: https://www.practicalpainmanagement.com/resources/ethics/can-call-myself-pain-specialist. Accessed October 30, 2021.

36. Peng P, Choiniere M, Dion D, et al. Challenges in accessing multidisciplinary pain treatment facilities in Canada. Can J Anaesth 2007;54(12):977–84.

37. Sokol RG, Pines R, Chew A. Multidisciplinary approach for managing complex pain and addiction in primary care: a qualitative study. Ann Fam Med 2021;19(3):224–31.

38. Martorella G, Kostic M, Lacasse A, et al. Knowledge, beliefs, and attitudes of emergency nurses toward people with chronic pain. SAGE Open Nurs 2019; 5. 2377960819871805.

39. Vijayaraghavan M, Penko J, Guzman D, et al. Primary care providers' views on chronic pain management among high-risk patients in safety net settings. Pain Med 2012;13(9):1141–8.

40. Patel SK, Gozal YM, Saleh MS, et al. Spinal cord stimulation failure: evaluation of factors underlying hardware explantation. J Neurosurg Spine 2019; 1–6.

41. Khan HA, Rabah NM, Winkelman RD, et al. The impact of preoperative depression on patient satisfaction with spine surgeons in the outpatient setting. Spine 2021;46(3):184–90.

42. Yang MMH, Riva-Cambrin J, Cunningham J, et al. Development and validation of a clinical prediction score for poor postoperative pain control following elective spine surgery. J Neurosurg Spine 2020; 1–10.

43. Kress HG, Aldington D, Alon E, et al. A holistic approach to chronic pain management that involves all stakeholders: change is needed. Curr Med Res Opin 2015;31(9):1743–54.

44. Cottrell E, Roddy E, Foster NE. The attitudes, beliefs and behaviours of GPs regarding exercise for chronic knee pain: a systematic review. BMC Fam Pract 2010;11:4.

45. Kumar K, Taylor RS, Jacques L, et al. Spinal cord stimulation versus conventional medical management for neuropathic pain: a multicentre randomised controlled trial in patients with failed back surgery syndrome. Pain 2007;132(1–2):179–88.

46. North RB, Kidd DH, Farrokhi F, et al. Spinal cord stimulation versus repeated lumbosacral spine surgery for chronic pain: a randomized, controlled trial. Neurosurgery 2005;56(1):98–106 [discussion: 106-107].

47. Deer TR, Pope JE, Lamer TJ, et al. The neuromodulation appropriateness consensus committee on best practices for dorsal root ganglion stimulation. Neuromodulation 2019;22(1):1–35.

48. Sweet JA, Mitchell LS, Narouze S, et al. Occipital nerve stimulation for the treatment of patients with medically refractory occipital neuralgia: congress of neurological surgeons systematic review and evidence-based guideline. Neurosurgery 2015; 77(3):332–41.

49. Petersen EA, Stauss TG, Scowcroft JA, et al. Effect of high-frequency (10-kHz) spinal cord stimulation in patients with painful diabetic neuropathy: a randomized clinical trial. JAMA Neurol 2021;78(6): 687–98.

50. Joshi GP, Beck DE, Emerson RH, et al. Defining new directions for more effective management of surgical pain in the United States: highlights of the inaugural Surgical Pain Congress. Am Surg 2014;80(3): 219–28.

51. Ljungqvist O, Scott M, Fearon KC. Enhanced Recovery After Surgery: a review. JAMA Surg 2017;152(3): 292–8.

52. Wick EC, Grant MC, Wu CL. Postoperative multimodal analgesia pain management with nonopioid analgesics and techniques: a review. JAMA Surg 2017;152(7):691–7.

53. Bartels K, Mayes LM, Dingmann C, et al. Opioid use and storage patterns by patients after hospital discharge following surgery. PloS one 2016;11(1): e0147972.

54. Elsarrag M, Soldozy S, Patel P, et al. Enhanced recovery after spine surgery: a systematic review. Neurosurg Focus 2019;46(4):E3.

55. Tong Y, Fernandez L, Bendo JA, et al. Enhanced recovery after surgery trends in adult spine surgery: a systematic review. Int J Spine Surg 2020;14(4): 623–40.

56. Wang MY, Chang P, Grossman J. Development of an enhanced recovery after surgery (ERAS) approach for lumbar spinal fusion. J Neurosurg Spine 2017; 26(4):411–8.

57. Dietz N, Sharma M, Adams S, et al. Enhanced recovery after surgery (ERAS) for spine surgery: a systematic review. World Neurosurg 2019;130: 415–26.

58. Corniola MV, Meling TR, Tessitore E. Enhanced recovery after spine surgery-a multinational survey assessing surgeons' perspectives. Acta Neurochir (Wien) 2020;162(6):1371–7.

59. Hunter CW, Stovall B, Chen G, et al. Anatomy, pathophysiology and interventional therapies for chronic pelvic pain: a review. Pain Physician 2018;21(2): 147–67.

60. Dun EC, Morozov V, Lakhi NA. Multidisciplinary approach to chronic pelvic pain. J Neurol Exp Neurosci 2015;1(1):1–5.

61. Passavanti MB, Pota V, Sansone P, et al. Chronic pelvic pain: assessment, evaluation, and objectivation. Pain Res Treat 2017;2017:9472925.

62. Roy H, Offiah I, Dua A. Neuromodulation for pelvic and urogenital pain. Brain Sci 2018;8(10).

63. Bridger C, Prabhala T, Dawson R, et al. Neuromodulation for chronic pelvic pain: a single-institution

experience with a collaborative team. Neurosurgery 2021;88(4):819–27.

64. Muller-Schwefe G, Jaksch W, Morlion B, et al. Make a CHANGE: optimising communication and pain management decisions. Curr Med Res Opin 2011; 27(2):481–8.

65. Upshur CC, Bacigalupe G, Luckmann R. They don't want anything to do with you": patient views of primary care management of chronic pain. Pain Med 2010;11(12):1791–8.

66. Meghani SH, Polomano RC, Tait RC, et al. Advancing a national agenda to eliminate disparities in pain care: directions for health policy, education, practice, and research. Pain Med 2012; 13(1):5–28.

67. Henssen D, Scheepers N, Kurt E, et al. Patients' expectations on spinal cord stimulation for failed back surgery syndrome: a qualitative exploration. Pain Pract 2018;18(4):452–62.

68. Joypaul S, Kelly F, McMillan SS, et al. Multi-disciplinary interventions for chronic pain involving education: a systematic review. PLoS one 2019;14(10): e0223306.

Health Care Disparity in Pain

Travis M. Hamilton, MD, Jared C. Reese, MD, Ellen L. Air, MD, PhD*

KEYWORDS

• Disparity • Pain • Race • Social determinants of health • Socioeconomics

KEY POINTS

- Socioeconomic factors, including race, income, and education, impact patients' health and treatment of disease.
- Non-whites and those of lower socioeconomic status experience a higher burden of chronic pain and relative undertreatment of that pain.
- Only by understanding these disparities and increasing the diversity of our health care workforce, can we improve the treatment of chronic pain.

INTRODUCTION

Health care disparities and their impact on the management of chronic pain are of increasing relevance in today's neurosurgical practice. Mounting literature on this subject has provided a better understanding of the relationship between socioeconomic status, racial, and ethnic disparities, and the management of chronic pain. It is generally known from multiple prior studies that a patient's sociodemographic profile influences the treatment of chronic pain, and many determinants of pain are affected by social conditions. This article describes several social determinants of health and how disadvantages in such categories affect chronic pain and neurosurgical outcomes. Significant progress can be made in the treatment of chronic pain by using evidence-based medicine and understanding the social factors that hinder optimal pain control.

The current literature and World Health Organization define social determinants of health as circumstances in which people are born, grow up, live, work, and age, and the systems put in place to deal with illness. In other words, factors such as age, gender, race, ethnicity, education, geographic location, culture, education, income, unemployment, transportation, literacy, and disability (to name a few) are a multifaceted list of risk factors that may influence a patient's health and their experience with health care systems. These variables are closely interrelated and complex, and it is difficult to isolate singular disparities for targeted study. Even so, any one factor may vary in significance from patient to patient. Although individual exposure to any of the aforementioned factors may be investigated, this article refers to the total collection of variables as one's respective socioeconomic status. Thus, an inequality in socioeconomic status between individuals, families, communities, populations, or global societies may be defined as a socioeconomic disparity. Given that many social factors contribute to disease, when differences arise between socioeconomic status as it relates to illness, this is referred to as a health care disparity.

RACE/ETHNICITY

Understanding the current landscape of disparities in pain management requires a look back at the roots of unequal care and the central role of race. An underpinning of slavery in the United States was the belief that black people are heartier with increased tolerance to pain.[1] Sadly, this false belief regarding biological differences remains prevalent in the general and medical community with a significant negative consequence to

Department of Neurosurgery, Henry Ford Hospital, 2799 West Grand Boulevard, Detroit, MI 48202, USA
* Corresponding author.
E-mail address: eair1@hfhs.org

Neurosurg Clin N Am 33 (2022) 251–260
https://doi.org/10.1016/j.nec.2022.02.003
1042-3680/22/© 2022 Elsevier Inc. All rights reserved.

neurosurgery.theclinics.com

individuals of color and management of their pain.[2] For example, racial bias has been shown to impede the timely diagnosis and treatment of diseases that typically present with painful conditions, such as cervical stenosis.[3] Data from the National Health Interview Survey (NHIS) and Center for Disease Control (CDC) show that Native Americans, Hispanic individuals, African American, and Mixed-race adults have substantially higher rates of activity limitations due to arthritis, osteoporosis, and chronic back conditions compared with White and Asian people in 2018[4] (**Fig. 1**). Despite the historical disproportion of pain in minority groups versus nonminority groups, pain complaints of individuals of color remain undertreated, particularly in the acute setting. For example, Lee and colleagues[5] demonstrated that there was no objective data to support that minority groups requested analgesics more or less than non-Hispanic white patients during emergency department visitations. Despite any evidence to support higher rates of opioid misuse in African Americans as compared with other ethnic groups, opioid use among African Americans tends to be more intensely monitored.[6]

There is evidence to suggest that there are racial differences in a patient's *experience and response to pain*. One study reported that African Americans are more sensitive to deep muscle pressure and mechanical pain, which was partially accounted for by increased pain catastrophizing. Black Americans endorse a higher and more debilitating degree of pain, and are subject to poorer outcomes after work-related injury and disability.[7,8] A lack of understanding about the social, psychological, and emotional response to pain may obscure one's proper recognition and treatment of a patient's painful experience.[6,9–11] As such, a lack of understanding of the historical frame of reference of the under-represented can also lead to the development of subconscious bias. The effect of implicit bias can have negative contributions to patient outcomes and lead to further unfair treatment and feelings of mistrust or wrongdoing.[12,13] In addition to patients' apparent sentiment of being undertreated, any additional societal loss associated with pain, injury, or disability from pain disorders such as trauma, arthritis, and fibromyalgia can be characterized as perceived injustice.[14,15] In a small sample population of 137 participants in the Southwest United States, Trost and colleagues demonstrated that Black Americans reported higher levels of perceived injustice related to chronic low back pain compared with white and Hispanic Americans, as well as higher pain intensity compared with Whites. Further validating this sentiment, a large retrospective cohort study

of 1,244,927 patients by Jones and colleagues[16] reported all minority ethnicities were significantly less likely to receive spinal cord stimulation (SCS) placement compared with White patients. In a recent systematic review by Morales and colleagues,[6] minority groups including Hispanic and African Americans have poorer outcomes and management of chronic pain compared with non-Hispanic Whites. This racial bias in the treatment of acute pain has also been extended to the pediatric populations as well.[17] From this, we see that a lack of cultural and racial sensitivity can influence the appropriate recognition and treatment of pain in the under-represented patient population.

A less-discussed dynamic of racial and ethnic disparity is the impact of culture and language. An individual's perception of pain can be greatly influenced by deeply rooted fundamental ethnic and cultural differences in the experience and communication of pain (eg, stigma, stoicism, machismo).[5,18,19,20] The influence of cultural factors are likely under-recognized. For example, Arab Americans are not represented on most national databases and questionnaires, as they often identify as White on national registries, obscuring nuances that may be important to optimal health care.[21,22]

Although some aspects of racial disparity and health equity have improved over the past 25 years (black-white gap), issues such as health justice and income disparities have worsened over time.[23] There continues to be a persistent disparity in the United States related to race despite the increasing body of published evidence and awareness describing this topic (**Fig. 2**). From a general health perspective, under-represented minorities in the United States experience systemic, social, and environmental factors that contribute to overall poor health status. Structural forces have evolved over the history of the United States that inhibit racial equality in health care such as pollution inequality, food insecurity/low access to healthy foods, mass incarceration, housing restrictions/redlining, educational attainment, family income, and life expectancy.[24] These societal influences can have a dramatic impact on the recognition, treatment, and long-term outcomes for patients with chronic pain.

SOCIOECONOMICS OF PAIN
Economics of Pain in Neurosurgery

The treatment of chronic pain is expensive. For example, common issues such as chronic low back pain and complex regional pain syndrome (CRPS) have an estimated annual cost of over

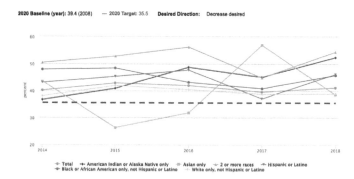

2020 Baseline (year): 39.4 (2008)   — 2020 Target: 35.5   **Desired Direction:** Decrease desired

-○- Total -+- American Indian or Alaska Native only -◇- Asian only -△- 2 or more races -▲- Hispanic or Latino
-◆- Black or African American only, not Hispanic or Latino --- White only, not Hispanic or Latino

Fig. 1. Adults with activity limitations due to arthritis (age-adjusted, percent, 18+ years) by race/ethnicity from 2014 to 2018 from the National Health Interview Survey (NHIS), CDC/NCHS,[4] 2020). (*Data Source*: National Health Interview Survey (NHIS); Centers for Disease Control and Prevention, National Center for Health Statistics (CDC/NCHS) Additional footnotes may apply to these data. Please refer to footnotes below the data table for further information).

$100 to 635 billion in the United States.[3,25] A comprehensive overview of US nonfederal community hospitals by Lad and colleagues demonstrated a progressive increase in hospital charges for SCS surgery over a 14-year period, totaling $215 million in 2006.[26] In this study, the average number of patients receiving SCS placement was stable; between approximately 3500 and 4500 cases per year and consistent with current data available through the Healthcare Cost and Utilization Project.[27] Approximately 32,000 SCS trial procedures were performed in 2006, and 10,000 permanent implants were placed based on a 3:1 trial to implant ratio.[26] As this datum is limited to inpatient procedures, it only represents a small fraction of the total number of SCS cases performed—noting that outpatient procedures are tenfold in number.[26] This trend coincides with recent reports of 10,762 SCS performed in a single state in 2018.[28] In 2020, the FDA estimates over 50,000 SCS are placed per year.[29]

Insurance

Recent studies by Labaran and colleagues[30] in 2020 report a range of 5.2 to 14.5 per 100,000 of all insurance beneficiaries underwent paddle SCS placement between 2007 and 2014 at a progressively increasing rate among most US territories. The Department of Health and Human Services' National Pain Strategy has recognized the economic utility, cost-benefit, and cost-efficiency of SCS placement and has urged insurers to allow for greater access to the nonopioid/prescription modality.[25,31]

As national registries and insurance companies are able to categorize patient information, several studies have uncovered insurance and payer disparities. Based on the information obtained from the National Inpatient Sample (from 2011 to 2015), Orhurhu and colleagues noted that patients with CRPS with private insurance had a statistically significant higher rate of SCS therapy utilization of 2.9% compared to patients with Medicare of 0.8% (*P* < .001). Patients with failed back surgery syndrome showed a similar trend, and patients with Medicaid and Self-payers had lower odds of SCS therapy compared with Medicare (OR = 0.50, *P* < .001).[32] This trend is also noted in prior reports.[33,34] The authors note that insurance payout is a contributing factor in SCS placement, particularly with government-sponsored insurance policies. However, opposite findings were identified by Labaran and colleagues[30], who demonstrated the annual adjusted rate of SCS placement (from 2007 to 2014) was highest among Medicare patients (5.9–17.5 per 100,000, *P* < .001) compared with private payers (5.2–14.5

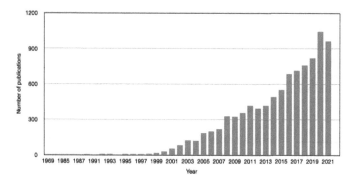

Fig. 2. Year and number of publications on "Racial disparities in healthcare". Pubmed accessed 10/10/2021.

per 100,000, $P < .001$) across all time points. In this study, 2 independent health insurance patient databases were used: private-payer insurance and Medicare, only evaluating patients undergoing open-laminectomy for SCS paddle placement. The authors concluded that this trend was observed because Medicare patients tended to be older with more advanced disease, warranting the need for SCS as a conservative, cost-effective treatment strategy with greater insurance coverage propensity. The limitation to truly uncover the disparities that exist with regards to insurance status is the use of publicly available databases that can only evaluate inpatient data. Other large, privately owned insurance databases can be accessible for research purposes but may not include information from all other private insurance companies or limitations may exist on obtaining nationwide data.

Education

Socioeconomic status builds on the complex interplay of demographic factors including education status. As such, education has been used as a surrogate for socioeconomic status. Within the neurosurgical literature, one's level of education has been shown to be inversely proportional to morbidity and mortality of several chronic diseases.[35–38] Over 50% of adults with less than a high-school education have activity limitations due to chronic pain and arthritis[39], which is significantly higher than that the percent of those with a 4-year college degree (approximately 35% per the NHIS and CDC in 2018 [**Fig. 3**]). Patient outcomes are influenced by the interplay between biopsychosocial and environmental factors. A cohort study by Roth and colleagues[38] demonstrated that the cognitive interpretation of pain as a signal of harm and catastrophizing were each independently associated with lower educational attainment and increased perceived disability secondary to chronic pain. This study found no associations between education and pain intensity, severity, or affective distress, but described the inverse association to self-reported disability. Other environmental associations between low education and chronic back pain include common modifiable risk factors (smoking and obesity) and increased risk for occupational hazards such as physical demand and work-related injuries, further confounding outcomes in this population.[40,41]

Income

Family income, another proxy for socioeconomic status, also tracks inversely with the prevalence of chronic pain.[37,42] In 2018, more than 60% of the US population with activity limitation due to chronic pain were below 100% of the poverty threshold. Bor and colleagues showed that the income-survival gradient across the United States has become more prevalent over time, further exacerbated by the effects of smoking, obesity, underutilization of medical care, and increased substance abuse/self-harm in patients with lower socioeconomic status.[43] Over the past decade, the income inequality gap has become more prevalent[23] (**Fig. 4**). Portenoy and colleagues[44] demonstrated the predictive association between low income and less educated patients with predicted pain disability. Data collection regarding income in clinic and hospital settings are limited and are often omitted as they are often self-reported or otherwise unattainable.[13,45] For example, some studies have attempted to use city boundaries using zip-codes as a surrogate for income level; however, this can lead to sampling error and reporting bias.[43] Yet, the literature suggests that overall neighborhood socioeconomic status is more predictive of pain than race/ethnicity.[46] A systematic review by Karran and colleagues[47] showed that income was independently linked to the increased prevalence and worse functional outcomes for patients with chronic low back pain. Jones and colleagues[16] noted in the largest and most recent retrospective trial to date on socioeconomic inequalities in SCS therapy that despite over a decade of literature validating the effect of disparities, little progress has been made.

There are several societal and systemic variables that contribute to the poor response to treatment within the lower socioeconomic population, such as the cost of prescriptions and outpatient follow-up.[37,48,49] In a cross-sectional study by Whitley and colleagues[50], lower income was associated with lower pain self-efficacy (perceived ability to function normally despite chronic pain) and coping self-efficacy strategies (perceived ability to manage chronic pain and cope with symptoms). There is substantial evidence to suggest other determinants of socioeconomic status such as a lack of access to financial resources, quality insurance, transportation, and social support are linked to low health literacy.[51–56] Although low health literacy is associated with a higher rate of mortality and morbidity for many chronic health conditions, recent systematic reviews suggest there is a significant lack of evidence specifically associating health literacy and chronic low back pain.[52,57] In addition, occupational status may not be a reliable indicator as those who are socioeconomically disadvantaged are more likely to be in physically demanding jobs with fewer accommodations.[37] Further research overcoming the statistical gaps

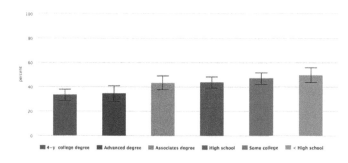

Fig. 3. Adults with activity limitation due to arthritis (age-adjusted, percent, 18+ years) by educational attainment in 2018 from the National Health Interview Survey (NHIS), CDC/NCHS.,[14] 2020). Error Bar (I) represents the 95% confidence interval. (*Data Source*: National Health Interview Survey (NHIS), CDC/NCHS.)

in data collection is still crucial to truly understand the mechanisms underlying financial disparities that can have a meaningful impact on patient outcomes.

CURRENT THERAPIES AND DISPARITIES
The Effect of COVID-19 on Disparity

The combination of governmental and social restrictions has exacerbated disparities in the treatment of chronic pain during the COVID pandemic.[58] Coincidentally, over 80% of chronic pain patients have independent associations with common risk factors for COVID-19, such as hypertension, diabetes, and depression.[59,60] Untreated chronic pain, particularly in groups associated with additional high-risk factors such as older age, contributes to systemic immunocompromise.[58] Social distancing exacerbated barriers to accessing proper medical care, such as scheduling appointments, transportation issues, cancellation of elective procedures, and clinician redeployment.[61] Karos and colleagues also noted that quarantining with family members can lead patients to minimize their pain to mitigate their perceived burden on their family members. Family

members also become desensitized to the pain of those they live with.[61] So not only is the emotional expression of pain not effectively communicated, but limitations on social activity add another barrier to treatment.[62] Chronic stress in systemically marginalized groups with poor access to care, financial strain, and language barriers has also played a significant role. Issues such as job security and unemployment along with an increase in domestic violence during the pandemic negatively impact the emotional well-being of patients with pain.[61]

Chronic pain is highly associated with mental health issues and substance abuse, both of which have been intensified by the COVID pandemic. Webster and colleagues[63] noted the widening of the inequality gap between these patients and the rest of society as their fear of stigmatization and injustice of their mental conditions became worse with social restriction, further fragmentation of individualized care, and cancellation of elective cases. Telehealth has offered a partial solution, allowing patients with increased family/home-related responsibilities (particularly women) to seek further medical treatment. Remote video

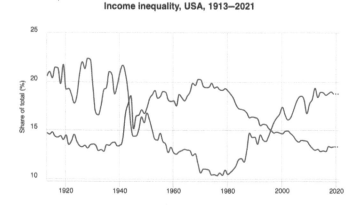

Fig. 4. Income inequality based on pretax national income for top 1% and bottom 50% of adults in the United States, between 1913 and 2020. Graph provided by www.wid.world.

patient encounters have offered a viable solution to the continuation of medical management of pain as well as treatment for opioid addiction.[58] However, this modality excludes patients in lower socioeconomic groups without access to such technology, or individuals fail to meet today's standard to technological literacy.[61,64]

Eliminating Disparities

There is undeniable evidence that societal and economic differences play a major role in the reporting, diagnosis, and treatment of patients with chronic pain. The underlying mechanisms are complicated and multifactorial. The key to addressing health inequity in pain management requires a fundamental understanding of the institutional effects of race, income, education, and culture, as well as the clinical and psychological impact of exacerbated pain, injustice, and bias from both the patient and clinician's point of view.

While we focused on the most studied causes of disparity in this review, there are several other marginalized groups that are burdened by unique societal restrictions and subjugated to biased and impartial care. Craig and colleagues[65] identified these individuals that are: (1) homeless, (2) torture survivors, (3) indigenous North Americans, (4) members of the LGBTQS2 communities, (5) refugees, (6) patients with human immunodeficiency disorder (HIV), and (7) Black veterans. These groups are often exposed to fear, violence, improper sleep and nutrition, and inadequate access to care. Alleviating disparity starts with proper identification, collection of population-level data, education among patients and clinicians, and implementation of sustainable outreach programs for patients and future clinicians. Fiscelle and colleagues[45] recommended 5 principles for addressing disparity issues from a health system perspective.

The first principle established by Fiscelle and colleagues is clearly defining and identifying the socioeconomic issue. Although there is extensive literature describing the impact and poor outcomes of health care inequity, it is clear that the complexity of the issue, with deep roots in the organizational structure and culture of America, will continually evolve. The second principle lies within the valid and appropriate means to collect data. Within each marginalized group is additional disparity related to comprehensive collection of data. Most of these issues lie in the difficulty of obtaining the data, such as lack of access to large privately owned databases and insurance data, language and geographic barriers, homelessness, and ethnicities that are not accurately accounted

for on hospital records or surveys. Galinskey and colleagues[66] demonstrated the possibility of capturing comprehensive interview data from Native Hawaiians and Pacific Islanders with the combination of using the American Community Survey as a framework and implementing multifaceted community engagement efforts in this difficult to survey population. The third principle involves the active use of quality measures stratified by race/ethnicity and socioeconomic position. This would allow for the reliable identification of high-risk patients to include for screening and advanced procedures. To allow for more meaningful and accurate comparisons between groups on a population level, the fourth principle calls for the adjustment of population-wide performance measures to be stratified by race/ethnicity and socioeconomic status. Lastly, reimbursement for the disadvantaged should be taken into consideration. These plans would aim to lower the current economic burden of health inequality in the United States, estimated at $230 billion.[67]

From the clinician-oriented perspective, there are ongoing programs designed to combat the disparity gap. Goree and colleagues[68] outlined a three-pronged approach to combat disparities individually directed toward patients, physicians, and outreach programs. Patient-centered outreach has been shown to increase the diagnosis, treatment rates, and outcomes of patients with breast, prostate, and colon cancer. The outreach efforts implemented are community-based and include social media and online platforms. Physician outreach to educate colleagues in various subspecialties participating in pain management (Internal medicine, Anesthesiology, Neurology, Neurosurgery) on the efficacy of advanced therapies such as neuromodulation, radiofrequency ablation, and neuropathic pain medications. Lastly, the authors include pipeline education on clinician implicit bias recognition and its effects early in medical training. This approach also encourages large specialty-specific societies to organize outreach events including underrepresented minority youths.

In 2000, the US Department of Health and Human Services instituted *Healthy People 2010*[69] as a means to improve the overall health of Americans while combating health care inequity, with the assistance of The American Medical Association (AMA). The Commission to End Healthcare Disparities was created by the AMA in 2004 along with the addition of the National Hispanic Medical Association. The commission was retired in 2016, with ongoing efforts to bridge the gap in patient disparity as well as efforts to enhance diversity within the physician workforce.[70] As the 5th iteration since 1979, *Healthy People 2030*[71] continues to promote progress on public health issues.

SUMMARY

Diversity in pain medicine involves the complex interplay between many variables and social factors that contribute, in their own unique way, to a lower standard of care and ultimately a dynamic disparity. For each facet of a patient's preoperative and postoperative care that places them in an identifiable category, there will be a subset within that population that appears to be underserved. Furthermore, there are identifiable groups that have not been recognized, or appropriately documented that make patient advocacy more challenging and difficult to track their outcomes. The implementation of community programs, publication of patient risk and outcomes, and education of the physician champions to combat these issues are necessary in educational/training programs and beyond to continue to bridge the disparity gap. As the social, political, and environmental climate continues to change, this field of work will also continue to evolve and adapt to new challenges.

Health care inequality must be recognized as an ongoing systemic disease. The future direction of disparity identification and mitigation should require the primary investigators to not only objectively examine the particular group of interest but also emphasize the limitations for the groups that could not be identified or were subject to exclusion. Only by recognizing the risk of data collection disparity can we begin to uncover potential opportunities to improve treatment. Despite the complex nature of health care inequity and the myriad of reports within the literature, the impact of racial and socioeconomic disparity remains prevalent. Despite active efforts to recruit a diverse body of clinicians, the physician population remains predominately white and male. However, there has been a significant increase in women and minorities in the youngest cohort of physicians, which portends a more diverse workforce in the future.[72] With the increase in public awareness of societal inequality, and less political stigmatization of racial and socioeconomic issues, there is an avenue to implement sustainable change. Health care inequality must be recognized as an issue of injustice, rather than a contributor to systemic disease. With improvements on data collection of groups that are difficult to capture statistically relevant information and sharing this information publicly, we can uncover the true effect and severity of pain as a disease.

CLINICS CARE POINTS

- Healthcare workers must recognize socioeconomic causes of disparity in pain management Undertreatment of pain increases overall burden of disease

DISCLOSURE

The authors have nothing to disclose.

REFERENCES

1. Cartwright S. Report on the diseases and physical peculiarities of the Negro race. New Orleans Med Surg J 1851;691–715.
2. Hoffman KM, Trawalter S, Axt JR, et al. Racial bias in pain assessment and treatment recommendations, and false beliefs about biological differences between blacks and whites. Proc Natl Acad Sci U S A 2016;113:4296–301. https://doi.org/10.1073/pnas.1516047113.
3. Elsamadicy AA, Yang S, Sergesketter AR, et al. Prevalence and cost analysis of complex regional pain syndrome (CRPS): a role for neuromodulation. Neuromodulation 2018;21:423–30. https://doi.org/10.1111/ner.12691.
4. Center for Disease Control, Healthy People, 2020, 2020 https://www.healthypeople.gov/2020/data/disparities/summary/Chart/4003/3.
5. Lee P, Le Saux M, Siegel R, et al. Racial and ethnic disparities in the management of acute pain in US emergency departments: Meta-analysis and systematic review. Am J Emerg Med 2019;37:1770–7. https://doi.org/10.1016/j.ajem.2019.06.014.
6. Morales ME, Yong RJ. Racial and ethnic disparities in the treatment of chronic pain. Pain Med 2021;22:75–90. https://doi.org/10.1093/pm/pnaa427.
7. Anderson KO, Green CR, Payne R. Racial and ethnic disparities in pain: causes and consequences of unequal care. J Pain 2009;10:1187–204. https://doi.org/10.1016/j.jpain.2009.10.002.
8. Trost Z, Sturgeon J, Guck A, et al. Examining injustice appraisals in a racially diverse sample of individuals with chronic low back pain. J Pain 2019;20:83–96. https://doi.org/10.1016/j.jpain.2018.08.005.
9. Edwards RR, Moric M, Husfeldt B, et al. Ethnic similarities and differences in the chronic pain experience: a comparison of african american, Hispanic, and white patients. Pain Med 2005;6:88–98. https://doi.org/10.1111/j.1526-4637.2005.05007.x.
10. Meints SM, Miller MM, Hirsh AT. Differences in pain coping between black and white americans: a meta-analysis. J Pain 2016;17:642–53. https://doi.org/10.1016/j.jpain.2015.12.017.

11. Meints SM, Wang V, Edwards RR. Sex and race differences in pain sensitization among patients with chronic low back pain. J Pain 2018;19:1461–70. https://doi.org/10.1016/j.jpain.2018.07.001.

12. Dehon E, Weiss N, Jones J, et al. A systematic review of the impact of physician implicit racial bias on clinical decision making. Acad Emerg Med 2017;24:895–904.   https://doi.org/10.1111/acem.13214.

13. Reinard K, Nerenz DR, Basheer A, et al. Racial disparities in the diagnosis and management of trigeminal neuralgia. J Neurosurg 2017;126:368–74. https://doi.org/10.3171/2015.11.JNS151177.

14. Sullivan MJL, Adams H, Horan S, et al. The role of perceived injustice in the experience of chronic pain and disability: scale development and validation. J Occup Rehabil 2008;18:249–61. https://doi.org/10.1007/s10926-008-9140-5.

15. Sullivan MJL, Scott W, Trost Z. Perceived injustice: a risk factor for problematic pain outcomes. Clin J Pain 2012;28:484–8. https://doi.org/10.1097/AJP.0b013e3182527d13.

16. Jones MR, Orhurhu V, O'Gara B, et al. Racial and socioeconomic disparities in spinal cord stimulation among the medicare population. Neuromodulation 2021;24:434–40. https://doi.org/10.1111/ner.13373.

17. Goyal MK, Kuppermann N, Cleary SD, et al. Racial disparities in pain management of children with appendicitis in emergency departments. JAMA Pediatr 2015;169:996–1002. https://doi.org/10.1001/jamapediatrics.2015.1915.

18. Booker SQ. African Americans' perceptions of pain and pain management: a systematic review. J Transcult Nurs 2016;27:73–80. https://doi.org/10.1177/1043659614526250.

19. Campbell CM, Edwards RR, Fillingim RB. Ethnic differences in responses to multiple experimental pain stimuli. Pain 2005;113:20–6. https://doi.org/10.1016/j.pain.2004.08.013.

20. Cancio R. Pain and masculinity: a cohort comparison between mexican american vietnam and post–9/11 combat veterans. Men and Masculinities 2020;23:725–48. https://doi.org/10.1177/1097184X18761779.

21. Campbell-Voytal KD, Schwartz KL, Hamade H, et al. Attitudes towards health research participation: a qualitative study of US Arabs and Chaldeans. Fam Pract 2019;36:325–31. https://doi.org/10.1093/fampra/cmy071.

22. National Archives and Records Administration. Revisions to the standards for the classification of federal data on Race and ethnicity. 2021 [WWW Document]. URL Available at: https://obamawhitehouse.archives.gov/omb/fedreg_1997standards. Accessed October 16, 2021.

23. Zimmerman FJ, Anderson NW. Trends in health equity in the United States by race/ethnicity, sex, and income, 1993-2017. JAMA Netw Open 2019;2:

e196386. https://doi.org/10.1001/jamanetworkopen.2019.6386.

24. Chandran M and Schulman K. Racial Disparities in Health and Healthcare. Health Services Research 57, 2022, 218–222, doi.org/10.1111/1475-6773.13957.

25. Hoelscher C, Riley J, Wu C, et al. Cost-effectiveness data regarding spinal cord stimulation for low back pain. Spine (Phila Pa 1976) 2017;42(Suppl 14):S72–9. https://doi.org/10.1097/BRS.0000000000002194.

26. Lad SP, Kalanithi PS, Arrigo RT, et al. Socioeconomic trends in spinal cord stimulation (SCS) surgery. Neuromodulation 2010;13:265–8. https://doi.org/10.1111/j.1525-1403.2010.00292.x.

27. Agency for Healthcare Research and Quality, 2021. Healthcare Cost and Utilization Project. [WWW Document] https://www.ahrq.gov/data/hcup/index.html.

28. Epstein RH, Dexter F, Podgorski EM, et al. Annual number of spinal cord stimulation procedures performed in the state of florida during 2018: implications for establishing neuromodulation centers of excellence. Neuromodulation 2019;13066. https://doi.org/10.1111/ner.13066.

29. FDA, 2020. Food and Drug Administration (FDA). Conduct a trial stimulation period before implanting a spinal cord stimulator (Scs) - letter to health care providers. [WWW Document] https://www.fda.gov/medical-devices/letters-health-care-providers/conduct-trial-stimulation-period-implanting-spinal-cord-stimulator-scs-letter-health-care-providers

30. Labaran L, Bell J, Puvanesarajah V, et al. Demographic trends in paddle lead spinal cord stimulator placement: private insurance and medicare beneficiaries. Neurospine 2020;17:384–9. https://doi.org/10.14245/ns.1938276.138.

31. US Department of Health and Human Services, 2016. Interagency Pain Research Coordinating Committee. National Pain Strategy: A Comprehensive Population Health-Level Strategy for Pain. [WWW Document] https://www.iprcc.nih.gov/sites/default/files/documents/NationalPainStrategy_508C.pdf

32. Orhurhu V, Gao C, Agudile E, et al. Socioeconomic disparities in the utilization of spinal cord stimulation therapy in patients with chronic pain. Pain Pract 2021;21:75–82. https://doi.org/10.1111/papr.12936.

33. Huang KT, Hazzard MA, Babu R, et al. Insurance disparities in the outcomes of spinal cord stimulation surgery. Neuromodulation 2013;16:428–34. https://doi.org/10.1111/ner.12059 [discussion: 434-435].

34. Missios S, Rahmani R, Bekelis K. Spinal cord stimulators: socioeconomic disparities in four US states. Neuromodulation 2014;17:451–5. https://doi.org/10.1111/ner.12101 [discussion: 455-456].

35. Dionne CE, Von Korff M, Koepsell TD, et al. Formal education and back pain: a review. J Epidemiol

Community Health 2001;55:455–68. https://doi.org/10.1136/jech.55.7.455.

36. Olson PR, Lurie JD, Frymoyer J, et al. Lumbar disc herniation in the spine patient outcomes research trial: does educational attainment impact outcome? Spine 2011;36:2324–32. https://doi.org/10.1097/BRS.0b013e31820bfb9a.

37. Poleshuck EL, Green CR. Socioeconomic disadvantage and pain. Pain 2008;136:235–8. https://doi.org/10.1016/j.pain.2008.04.003.

38. Roth RS, Geisser ME. Educational achievement and chronic pain disability: mediating role of pain-related cognitions. Clin J Pain 2002;18:286–96. https://doi.org/10.1097/00002508-200209000-00003.

39. Pincus T, Callahan LF, Burkhauser RV. Most chronic diseases are reported more frequently by individuals with fewer than 12 years of formal education in the age 18-64 United States population. J Chronic Dis 1987;40:865–74. https://doi.org/10.1016/0021-9681(87)90186-x.

40. Dionne C, Koepsell TD, Von Korff M, et al. Formal education and back-related disability. In Search of an explanation. Spine (Phila Pa 1976) 1995;20:2721–30. https://doi.org/10.1097/00007632-199512150-00014.

41. van Poppel MMN, Koes WB, Devillé W, et al. Risk factors for back pain incidence in industry: a prospective study. Pain 1998;77:81–6. https://doi.org/10.1016/S0304-3959(98)00085-2.

42. Shmagel A, Foley R, Ibrahim H. Epidemiology of chronic low back pain in US adults: data from the 2009-2010 National health and nutrition examination survey. Arthritis Care Res (Hoboken) 2016;68:1688–94. https://doi.org/10.1002/acr.22890.

43. Bor J, Cohen GH, Galea S. Population health in an era of rising income inequality: USA, 1980-2015. Lancet 2017;389:1475–90. https://doi.org/10.1016/S0140-6736(17)30571-8.

44. Portenoy RK, Ugarte C, Fuller I, et al. Population-based survey of pain in the United States: differences among white, African American, and Hispanic subjects. J Pain 2004;5:317–28. https://doi.org/10.1016/j.jpain.2004.05.005.

45. Fiscella K, Franks P, Gold MR, et al. Inequality in quality: addressing socioeconomic, racial, and ethnic disparities in health care. JAMA 2000;283:2579–84. https://doi.org/10.1001/jama.283.19.2579.

46. Fuentes M, Hart-Johnson T, Green CR. The association among neighborhood socioeconomic status, race and chronic pain in black and white older adults. J Natl Med Assoc 2007;99:1160–9.

47. Karran EL, Grant AR, Moseley GL. Low back pain and the social determinants of health: a systematic review and narrative synthesis. Pain 2020;161:2476–93. https://doi.org/10.1097/j.pain.0000000000001944.

48. Kennedy J, Morgan S. A cross-national study of prescription nonadherence due to cost: data from the Joint Canada-United States Survey of Health. Clin Ther 2006;28:1217–24. https://doi.org/10.1016/j.clinthera.2006.07.009.

49. Mukherjee S, Sullivan G, Perry D, et al. Adherence to treatment among economically disadvantaged patients with panic disorder. Psychiatr Serv 2006;57:1745–50. https://doi.org/10.1176/ps.2006.57.12.1745.

50. Whitley MD, Herman PM, Aliyev GR, et al. Income as a predictor of self-efficacy for managing pain and for coping with symptoms among patients with chronic low back pain. J Manipulative Physiol Ther 2021;44:433–44. https://doi.org/10.1016/j.jmpt.2021.05.004.

51. Briggs AM, Jordan JE. The importance of health literacy in physiotherapy practice. J Physiother 2010;56:149–51. https://doi.org/10.1016/S1836-9553(10)70018-7.

52. Dewalt D, Berkman N, Sheridan S, et al. Literacy and health outcomes: a systematic review of the literature. J Gen Intern Med 2004;19:1228–39. https://doi.org/10.1111/j.1525-1497.2004.40153.x.

53. Edward J, Carreon LY, Williams MV, et al. The importance and impact of patients' health literacy on low back pain management: a systematic review of literature. Spine J 2018;18:370–6. https://doi.org/10.1016/j.spinee.2017.09.005.

54. Jordan JE, Briggs AM, Brand CA, et al. Enhancing patient engagement in chronic disease self-management support initiatives in Australia: the need for an integrated approach. Med J Aust 2008;189:S9–13. https://doi.org/10.5694/j.1326-5377.2008.tb02202.x.

55. Kaplan GA, Salonen JT. Socioeconomic conditions in childhood and ischaemic heart disease during middle age. BMJ 1990;301:1121–3. https://doi.org/10.1136/bmj.301.6761.1121.

56. Sudore RL, Yaffe K, Satterfield S, et al. Limited literacy and mortality in the elderly: the health, aging, and body composition study. J Gen Intern Med 2006;21:806–12. https://doi.org/10.1111/j.1525-1497.2006.00539.x.

57. See YKC, Smith HE, et al. Health literacy and health outcomes in patients with low back pain: a scoping review. BMC Med Inform Decis Mak 2021;21:215. https://doi.org/10.1186/s12911-021-01572-0.

58. Puntillo F, Giglio M, Brienza N, et al. Impact of COVID-19 pandemic on chronic pain management: looking for the best way to deliver care. Best Pract Res Clin Anaesthesiol 2020;34:529–37. https://doi.org/10.1016/j.bpa.2020.07.001.

59. Barnett K, Mercer SW, Norbury M, et al. Epidemiology of multimorbidity and implications for health care, research, and medical education: a cross-sectional study. Lancet 2012;380:37–43. https://doi.org/10.1016/S0140-6736(12)60240-2.

60. van Hecke O, Hocking LJ, Torrance N, et al. Chronic pain, depression and cardiovascular disease linked through a shared genetic predisposition: analysis of

a family-based cohort and twin study. PLoS One 2017;12:e0170653. https://doi.org/10.1371/journal.pone.0170653.

61. Karos K, McParland JL, Bunzli S, et al. The social threats of COVID-19 for people with chronic pain. Pain 2020;161:2229–35. https://doi.org/10.1097/j.pain.0000000000002004.

62. Malhotra N, Kunal S. The catch-22 of the COVID-19 "lockdown. Adv Respir Med 2020;88:285–6. https://doi.org/10.5603/ARM.a2020.0097.

63. Webster F, Connoy L, Sud A, et al. Grappling with chronic pain and poverty during the COVID-19 pandemic. Can J Pain 2020;4:125–8. https://doi.org/10.1080/24740527.2020.1766855.

64. Seifert A, Cotten SR, Xie B. A double burden of exclusion? digital and social exclusion of older adults in times of COVID-19. J Gerontol B Psychol Sci Soc Sci 2021;76:e99–103. https://doi.org/10.1093/geronb/gbaa098.

65. Craig KD, Holmes C, Hudspith M, et al. Pain in persons who are marginalized by social conditions. Pain 2020;161:261–5. https://doi.org/10.1097/j.pain.0000000000001719.

66. Galinsky AM, Simile C, Zelaya CE, et al. Surveying strategies for hard-to-survey populations: lessons from the native hawaiian and pacific islander national health interview survey. Am J Public Health 2019;109:1384–91. https://doi.org/10.2105/AJPH.2019.305217.

67. Sarfraz A, Sarfraz Z, Barrios A, et al. Understanding and promoting racial diversity in healthcare settings to address disparities in pandemic crisis management. J Prim Care Community Health 2021;12. https://doi.org/10.1177/21501327211018354.

68. Goree J, Vanterpool S. The need for outreach in pain and neuroscience. American Society of Pain and Neuroscience; 2020.

69. Healthy People 2010. [WWW Document] https://www.cdc.gov/nchs/healthy_people/hp2010.htm

70. AMA. Strategies for Enhancing Diversity in the Physician Workforce H-200.951. American Medical Association; 2021.

71. Healthy People 2030. [WWW document] https://health.gov/healthypeople

72. AAMC. Diversity in medicine: facts and figures 2019. AAMC. 2019. Available at: https://www.aamc.org/data-reports/workforce/report/diversity-medicine-facts-and-figures-2019. Accessed October 29, 2021.

Nonopioid Postoperative Pain Management in Neurosurgery

Nathan A. Shlobin, BA, Joshua M. Rosenow, MD*

KEYWORDS

• Analgesia • Enhanced recovery after surgery • Opioid • Neurologic surgery • Spine surgery

KEY POINTS

- Nonopioid management of postoperative pain is essential to improve postneurosurgical pain while reducing the postoperative use of opioids.
- An array of preoperative, intraoperative, and postoperative medication-based strategies exists.
- Multimodal, multidisciplinary approaches incorporating medical therapies, lifestyle modifications, clinical practices, and psychological interventions may provide optimal benefit.
- Consideration of patient-specific factors and the best-available evidence for interventions lays the foundation for the development of these approaches.

INTRODUCTION

Postoperative pain after neurosurgery is common and more severe than many physicians and patients anticipate.[1–4] Approximately 60% of patients experience pain following craniotomy, two-thirds of whom experience pain of moderate to severe intensity.[1] Pain most frequently occurs and is most severe in the first 48 hours after surgery.[2] Additionally, postoperative pain management is often inadequate, compounding the overall burden to patients.[5,6] The postoperative experience of pain may be a combination of nociceptive, neuropathic, psychological, and behavioral components.[7] Generally, opioids remain a common first-line analgesic prescribed to neurosurgical patients, rooted in animal model studies that demonstrated that opioids reduce nociceptive pain via synergistic action at spinal and supraspinal sites.[8–10] Neurosurgical patients are often discharged on one or more opioid medications.[11] However, the use of strong opioids on neurosurgical wards has increased over time.[12]

Recent developments have encouraged efforts to minimize the use of opioids for postoperative neurosurgical pain. The association of opioid use with overdose deaths has highlighted the presence of an "opioid epidemic."[13,14] Tolerance and physical dependence may develop due to opioid activation of dorsal horn N-methyl-D-aspartate (NMDA) systems, inactivation of u-opioid receptors, upregulation of the cyclic adenosine monophosphate pathway, and spinal dynorphin release.[15–19] Opioids also have frequent side effects, including cognitive slowing, hyperalgesia, constipation, and vomiting.[15] Concerns regarding the efficacy of opioids in treating pain following neurosurgery continue to arise.[20] Opioids have also been associated with an array of unfavorable clinical and functional outcomes. Preoperative opioid use has been associated with increased postoperative opioid use, hospitalization duration, risk of revision, and health care costs and poorer return to work status following spine surgery.[21] Lastly, opioid use is now an object of social stigma in many regions.[22,23]

These developments have highlighted the need for nonopioid strategies for the management of postoperative pain in neurosurgical patients. In this article, we describe strategies to manage postoperative pain in neurosurgery, focusing on a variety of nonopioid interventions within the preoperative, intraoperative, and postoperative periods.

Department of Neurological Surgery, Northwestern University Feinberg School of Medicine, 676 North St. Clair Street, Suite 2210, Chicago, IL 60611, USA
* Corresponding author.
E-mail address: jrosenow@nm.org

Neurosurg Clin N Am 33 (2022) 261–273
https://doi.org/10.1016/j.nec.2022.02.004
1042-3680/22/© 2022 Elsevier Inc. All rights reserved.

PREOPERATIVE STRATEGIES

Preoperative pain management strategies seek to modify pain transmission before the surgical insult that causes pain.

Methadone

Methadone is a combined opiate receptor agonist and N-methyl-D-aspartate receptor antagonist with a long half-life (15–60 hours) used as a replacement opioid in therapy for opioid dependence due to its mitigation of opioid-mediated tolerance and hyperalgesia.[24] Methadone has been explored as an option to reduce postoperative opioid use when administered before incision. Gottschalk and colleagues[25] randomized 29 patients undergoing multilevel thoracolumbar spine surgery to receive 0.2 mg/kg of methadone before incision or 0.75 ug/kg loading dose with a 0.25 ug/kg/h continuous infusion of sufentanil intraoperatively. Methadone reduced postoperative opioid requirement by nearly 50% at 48 hours relative to sufentanil.[25] Pain scores as measured by visual-analog scale (VAS) were 50% lower in the methadone group compared with the sufentanil group at 48 hours following surgery.[25] Murphy and colleagues[26] conducted a double-blinded randomized controlled trial (RCT) in which 120 patients undergoing spinal fusion were randomized to 0.2 mg/kg of methadone at induction or 2 mg of hydromorphone at surgical closure. Median hydromorphone used was reduced through final evaluation during the night of postoperative day 3 in the methadone group, while pain scores at rest, with movement, and with coughing were lower in the methadone group in more than 70% of assessments.[26] Overall satisfaction was higher in the methadone group until the morning of postoperative day 3. The studies by Gottschalk and colleagues and Murphy and colleagues reported no difference in adverse events[25,26].

Gabapentinoids

Gabapentin and pregabalin, members of the gabapentinoid class that inhibit the alpha 2-delta subunit of voltage-gated calcium channels, were initially approved for seizures and some neuropathic pain but have been increasingly prescribed for nociceptive pain.[27–29] An early meta-analysis of gabapentin for any surgery demonstrated that a single preoperative oral dose of 1200 mg of gabapentin resulted in a mean reduction of VAS score of 10.87 mm and mean reduction in opioid use of 7.25 mg at 24 hours.[30] A meta-analysis of surgical studies, mostly examining preoperative gabapentin, by Clarke and colleagues[31] determined that

perioperative gabapentin was associated with a moderate-to-large reduction in the development of chronic postsurgical pain (>2-months postsurgery), while pregabalin was associated with a very large reduction. A systematic review of 97 studies with 7201 patients indicated that the overall 24-h morphine sparing effect was 5.8 mg. However, these systematic reviews have also shown that many included studies are a low evidence grade, with estimates of efficacy limited by bias and insufficient data, and that gabapentinoid use may be associated with a greater risk of adverse events.[32–34]

Studies specific to neurosurgery have demonstrated some promising results. A RCT of patients undergoing craniotomy for supratentorial tumor resection indicated that 1200 mg of gabapentin for 7 days before surgery and postoperatively decreased postoperative pain within the first hour postsurgery and analgesic consumption but was associated with delayed extubation and increased postoperative sedation.[35] A double-blinded, placebo-controlled RCT of patients undergoing suboccipital or subtemporal craniotomy determined that 600 mg of gabapentin the night before surgery and again 2 hours before anesthesia induction decreased postoperative pain scores at rest and with movement at 24 hours postoperatively as well as resulted in decreased postoperative vomiting, and mean consumption of intraoperative propofol and remifentanil.[36] Pain at 48 hours was not reduced significantly and gabapentin not only did not decrease overall postoperative opioid consumption but was associated with increased postoperative sedation.[36] Another trial determined that twice-daily 150 mg pregabalin attenuated preoperative anxiety and improved sleep quality, reduced postoperative pain scores and analgesic usage, without increased adverse events.[37] An early meta-analysis of 7 trials demonstrated that gabapentin and pregabalin reduced postoperative narcotic consumption relative to placebo in the first day after lumbar surgery.[38] A more recent series of 86 patients by Urban and colleagues[39] reported no advantage in terms of postoperative intravenous (IV) narcotic usage, physical therapy milestones, or length of stay among patients undergoing lumbar fusion who received pregabalin. However, the dose of pregabalin was 150 mg 1 hour before surgery and then 150 mg daily, which is lower than that used in other studies.[39]

INTRAOPERATIVE STRATEGIES

Intraoperative pain management seeks to reduce the activation of pain responses while tissue injury is occurring.

Local Anesthetic Infiltration

Numerous studies have examined the utility of local anesthetic infiltration before incision, intraoperatively, before wound closure, or immediately following wound closure. Common agents are bupivacaine, ropivacaine, and lidocaine. Meta-analyses in other surgical fields have demonstrated the utility of local anesthetic infiltration in decreasing postoperative pain.[40,41]

Studies within neurosurgery have generally shown favorable results for preincision local anesthetic. An RCT found that preemptive scalp infiltration with 0.5% ropivacaine and 1% lidocaine delays time to demand for postoperative analgesics and reduces postoperative morphine consumption.[42] However, another RCT indicated that preincision infiltration with 25 mL of 0.25% bupivacaine did not decrease postcraniotomy pain and analgesic requirement but did delay time to the requirement of first analgesic dose.[43] A retrospective study of patients undergoing unilateral lumbar laminectomy reported that perineural lidocaine infiltration immediately following exposure promoted longer time to first postoperative analgesia request and required less analgesic overall.[44] A meta-analysis of 11 RCTs determined that spinal intramuscular local anesthetic infiltration prior to wound closure reduces postoperative opioid requirements and reduces pain at 1-h postsurgery but not necessarily at 12 or 24 hours.[45] Another RCT determined that preclosure spinal muscle infiltration with bupivacaine or levobupivacaine promoted effective pain control with reduced opioid consumption for patients undergoing unilateral lumbar laminectomy.[46] However, a systematic review of RCTs examining wound infiltration with local analgesics in spinal surgery determined that the reduction in pain intensity and opioid consumption was between 8 and 40 mm on a 100 mm VAS in a minority of studies, with no difference in the remainder of studies.[47] Using a different approach, Yörükoglu, and colleagues[48] conducted an RCT of a combination of low-dose intrathecal and epidural morphine and found that this intervention resulted in lower postoperative pain scores and early analgesic requirement with no increase in side effects compared with paraspinal bupivacaine. The addition of clonidine to local bupivacaine infiltration has also been shown to prolong postoperative analgesia in posterior lumbar spine surgeries.[49] Local anesthetic injected around scalp nerves is superior for early pain relief when injected after surgery and for late pain relief when injected before surgery, likely due to the blockade of the afferent barrage that occurs at the time of surgical incision.[50] Law-

Koune and colleagues[51]. determined that scalp infiltration with bupivacaine or ropivacaine immediately following skin closure decreased morphine consumption during the first 2 postoperative hours after craniotomy in their RCT.

Scalp Block

Scalp block is a regional anesthesia technique that is more extensive than simple wound infiltration. A prospective placebo-controlled RCT determined that scalp block with 0.5% bupivacaine immediately before pin holder application decreased pain intensity to a greater degree compared with local anesthetic infiltration.[52] Both methods reduced morphine consumption within the first postoperative day.[52] An RCT of 80 patients scheduled for stereotactic brain biopsy determined that scalp block with 0.5% bupivacaine reduced pain during the fixation of the stereotactic frame and skin incision. The block also reduced the need for further local anesthetic infiltration compared with simple local subcutaneous infiltration and promoted lower pain intensity and reduced headache incidence postoperatively.[53] Chaki and colleagues[54] found that scalp block with a mixture of lidocaine and ropivacaine was an effective and safe mode of analgesia in patients undergoing awake craniotomy. These studies corroborate the results of an earlier meta-analysis of 7 RCTs that indicated that regional scalp block preoperatively or postoperatively reduced pain scores and opioid requirements postsurgery.[55] However, a retrospective study of patients undergoing deep brain stimulation indicated that dose of analgesics did not differ during and after surgery between patients receiving scalp block and simple local anesthetic.[56] Another recent trial has demonstrated that bilateral scalp blocks using bupivacaine with epinephrine near the close of surgery did not reduce mean postoperative VAS score, overall opioid consumption at 24 hours, or time-to-discharge from the postanesthesia care unit or hospital.[57] However, it may not be surprising that scalp blocks at the end of surgery (after the surgical insult has already occurred) may not be very effective at reducing postoperative pain.[58]

Steroids

Multiple studies have examined the effect of intraoperative steroids on postoperative pain, often in conjunction with local anesthetics. One study of patients undergoing microdiscectomy determined that patients receiving intramuscular methylprednisolone acetate and IV methylprednisolone sodium succinate in addition to bupivacaine infiltration into paraspinal musculature at skin incision and closure required less postoperative narcotic analgesia and more frequently reported complete relief of back or radicular pain relative to those who received bupivacaine alone or those receiving neither bupivacaine nor steroids.[59] Mirzai and colleagues[60] randomly assigned patients to receive 0.25% bupivacaine injection during wound closure with the placement of autologous fat soaked in methylprednisolone over the exposed nerve root or to saline placebo. The intervention decreased meperidine usage, with no difference in VAS scores between the groups.[60] An RCT demonstrated that local methylprednisolone applied to nerve roots with 0.375% bupivacaine wound infiltration was associated with lower postoperative pain and cumulative morphine dose relative to a placebo.[61] Another RCT found improvement in pain scores at postoperative day 1, mean 24-hour opioid requirement, and mean inpatient stay in patients who had triamcinolone acetonide and bupivacaine instilled into the nerve root relative to controls, with no difference in pain score at 8 weeks postoperatively.[62] Meta-analyses have also demonstrated promising results. A meta-analysis of 1933 patients undergoing lumbar discectomy demonstrated that intraoperative epidural steroids reduced pain, decreased hospital stay, and improved neurologic status, with no effect on infection rates.[63] A meta-analysis of patients undergoing lumbar surgery determined that intraoperative epidural steroids improved pain control, reduced postoperative opioid use, and reduced length of stay.[64] Triamcinolone and dexamethasone performed similarly, while methylprednisolone performed worse at 24 hours.[64]

Methadone

The use of methadone has extended from preoperative to intraoperative settings. In their systematic review of 13 trials, Machado determined that intraoperative methadone administration decreased pain at rest and movement to an extent greater than other opioids up to 48 hours after surgery and decreased postoperative opioid consumption.[65] A meta-analysis of 10 studies by D'Souza and colleagues[66] determined that patients receiving methadone generally had lower postoperative pain scores and greater satisfaction with analgesia, with no difference in time-to-extubation, time-to-analgesia request, length of stay, or complications. However, there are risks. In a study of 1478 adult patients undergoing elective spinal fusion of at least 2 levels, Dunn and colleagues[67] reported mild to moderate respiratory depression following one dose of intraoperative

methadone, necessitating monitoring postoperatively.

Ketamine

Ketamine, an NMDA receptor antagonist, has also been shown to improve pain control. A Cochrane review demonstrated that intraoperative ketamine reduced pain, nausea, vomiting, and use of opioids following surgery.[68] Loftus and colleagues[69] conducted RCT of opiate-dependent patients undergoing lumbar spine surgery for which the treatment group received 0.5 mg/kg IV ketamine on induction and continuous infusion of 10 mcg/kg/min until wound closure. The authors reported total morphine consumption was reduced in the treatment groups at 24 hours, 48 hours, and 6 weeks after the procedure, with reported pain intensity also reduced at 6 weeks.[69] Two RCTs on spinal fusion have demonstrated reduced morphine and hydromorphone consumption up to 24 hours after spinal fusion surgery in opioid-dependent patients.[70,71] Given that ketamine does not increase intracranial pressure to the same extent as do intraoperative opioids, ketamine may also be an alternative to opioids for certain cranial surgeries.[72] Further studies are required.

Acetaminophen

Acetaminophen has been increasingly studied as an opioid alternative after neurosurgery, especially since the introduction of IV formulations. A meta-analysis of surgical trials demonstrated that IV or oral acetaminophen combined with patient-controlled analgesia (PCA) morphine reduced postoperative consumption of morphine relative to PCA morphine alone but not the incidence of morphine-related adverse effects.[73] Trials within cranial surgery have demonstrated promising, but not convincing, results. In their blinded RCT, Sivakumar randomized 204 cranial surgery patients to 1000 mg IV acetaminophen every 8 hours for 48 hours, with the first dose provided intraoperatively after the conclusion of the procedure, or a normal saline placebo.[74] Patients in the acetaminophen group experienced lower postoperative pain.[74] However, this study and others examining cranial surgery have found no difference in overall opioid consumption postoperatively and no difference in opioid-related adverse effects.[74–76] Nevertheless, craniotomy patients who receive IV acetaminophen have reported greater satisfaction with overall postoperative pain management.[76] A recent meta-analysis of 5 RCTs determined that IV acetaminophen was associated with decreased postoperative pain, need for rescue analgesics, and analgesic doses following craniotomy.[77] Studies within spine surgery have demonstrated conflicting results. A nationwide database study demonstrated that IV acetaminophen reduced inpatient opioid use with reduced odds for opioid-associated adverse outcomes.[78] However, an RCT found IV acetaminophen of 90 mg/kg/d as an adjuvant to oxycodone improved analgesia but did not reduce oxycodone consumption during 24 hours after spine surgery in pediatric patients.[79] However, another study found that IV acetaminophen after spinal surgery was associated with lower opioid doses, improved discharge status, lower resource use, and lower costs relative to oral acetaminophen.[80]

Ketorolac

Ketorolac, a nonselective cyclooxygenase inhibitor and first-generation nonsteroidal anti-inflammatory drug (NSAID), has also been studied. One series demonstrated that ketorolac is as safe as diclofenac and ketoprofen for pain relief after major surgery.[81] Le Roux and Samudrala reported that ketorolac in combination with opioids was more effective than opioids alone in managing postoperative pain following lumbar disc surgery and was associated with shorter hospitalization.[82] Another study found that IV bolus ketorolac on surgical closure and then every 6 hours for 36 hours along with morphine PCA reduced postoperative pain more effectively than morphine PCA alone following lumbar disc surgery.[83] Other randomized studies have demonstrated that ketorolac results in improved analgesia, decreased morphine consumption, and decreased somnolence when used as an adjunct to morphine PCA.[84,85] Using ketorolac 7.5 mg every 6 hours has a morphine-sparing effect in patients undergoing spine stabilization surgery equivalent to that of larger doses.[85] A retrospective study found that wound infiltration with levobupivacaine, ketorolac, and epinephrine led to reductions in overall pain, consumption of morphine, use of PCA, and length of stay.[86] However, an RCT found that neither ketorolac nor bupivacaine decreased postoperative narcotic use in patients who underwent microsurgical lumbar discectomy.[87] Increased risk of hemorrhage is a common concern with the use of ketorolac intraoperatively or postoperatively in neurosurgical patients. However, in their retrospective review of 1451 pediatric patients undergoing craniotomy, Richardson and colleagues[88] reported no differences in clinically significant or insignificant hemorrhage between patients who received ketorolac postoperatively and those who did not. A nested case-control study also failed to find an association with ketorolac use and symptomatic bleeding requiring surgery.[89] Another concern is fusion rates after spine surgery. Although somewhat equivocal, the existing base of evidence indicates that ketorolac use after spine surgery may be safe, particularly when normal doses of ketorolac are used for less than 14 days.[90–93]

Liposomal Bupivacaine

Liposomal bupivacaine, composed of bupivacaine loaded into multivesicular liposomes, theoretically increases the duration of local anesthetic action by slowing the release of bupivacaine and delays peak plasma concentrations for up to 96 to 120 hours.[94] In their case-control study of 116 patients, Grieff and colleagues determined that postoperative opioid requirements after posterior spinal decompression surgery were approximately 50% lower in the group receiving liposomal bupivacaine into the paraspinal muscles compared with the standard bupivacaine group,[95] though this difference was not significant.[96] One retrospective cohort study demonstrated that liposomal bupivacaine reduced pain scores, narcotic equivalents, and length of stay relative to nonliposomal local anesthetic in patients undergoing transforaminal lumbar interbody fusion, while another retrospective study determined liposomal bupivacaine in lumbar interbody fusion decreased length of stay but did not reduce pain or opioid use within 3 days postoperatively.[97] A study of pediatric patients undergoing Chiari I malformation surgery reported reduced pain scores and opioid use for patients receiving liposomal bupivacaine within the first 24 hours postoperatively but no difference beyond that time period.[98] Given these results, further larger RCTs may be needed to definitively delineate the potential utility of liposomal bupivacaine in neurosurgical patients.

Dexmedetomidine

Dexmedetomidine, a selective alpha-2 adrenoreceptor agonist with sympatholytic, sedative, amnestic, and analgesic properties, but without respiratory depression, has been increasingly used for pain control.[99] Multiple meta-analyses have demonstrated the utility of dexmedetomidine in decreasing postoperative pain and exerting opioid-sparing effects, including decreased nausea and vomiting and quicker recovery.[100–103] An RCT found that dexmedetomidine reduced pain, tramadol consumption, and postoperative nausea and vomiting in craniotomy patients relative to placebo.[104] Another study determined that dexmedetomidine infusion at 0.5 ug/kg for 10 minutes then at 0.3 ug/kg/h until closing plus sufentanil improved pain scores and reduced postoperative opioid consumption and related adverse effects without increasing sedation.[105] A meta-analysis of 11 RCTs including 674 neurosurgical patients found that dexmedetomidine reduced perioperative pain intensity and perioperative and postanesthesia care unit opioid consumption.[106] A more recent meta-analysis of 22 RCTs of 1348 patients undergoing craniotomy determined that there was moderate to high quality evidence demonstrating reduced postoperative pain, nausea and vomiting, hypertension, and tachycardia when comparing dexmedetomidine to placebo, with moderate quality evidence indicating no difference in these outcomes.[107] Moderate quality evidence showed no difference in the proportion of craniotomies completed without serious complications or in postoperative pain when comparing dexmedetomidine to active comparators, including remifentanil, fentanyl, or propofol.[107] Intrathecal infusion of a combination of bupivacaine and dexmedetomidine has also been shown to be associated with prolonged postoperative analgesia.[108]

Awake Versus Asleep Surgery

As awake brain surgery becomes more commonly used, the effect of avoiding general anesthesia on postoperative analgesia must be considered. A recent retrospective study compared patients undergoing craniotomy for supratentorial intra-axial tumors awake under regional anesthesia versus under general anesthesia.[109] Patients in the regional anesthesia group reported less postoperative pain used lower doses of opioids after surgery.[109] Similarly, the time until opioids was requested for pain was greater in the regional anesthesia group, while somnolence was reduced.[109]

POSTOPERATIVE STRATEGIES

Postoperative pain management seeks to mitigate pain signaling following the conclusion of the surgery.

Wound Catheters with Continuous Subcutaneous Infusion

Wound catheters with continuous subcutaneous infusion pumps have been used in a variety of surgical fields due to their ability to provide a constant rate of local analgesia. A systematic review of surgical RCTs found that continuous postoperative local anesthetic infused via wound catheters improved pain control, reduced opioid use and side effects, decreased hospital stay, and

increased patient satisfaction.[110] A meta-analysis of 14 surgical RCTs indicated that continuous wound infusion with ropivacaine promoted improved pain outcomes and reduced opioid use relative to placebo.[111]

Subcutaneous anesthetic infusion has also been used in neurosurgery with favorable. One RCT of patients undergoing cervical laminectomy determined that bilateral subfascial continuous 0.5% bupivacaine infusion at 2 mg/h for 3 postoperative days via an epidural catheter improved pain, reduced narcotic use, and promoted early ambulation with no serious adverse events relative to placebo.[112] A retrospective study demonstrated that continuous wound infiltration with ropivacaine promoted reduced pain, reduced PCA requirement, and improved patient satisfaction.[113] However, another RCT of posterior spinal fusion patients determined that continuous wound infiltration with ropivacaine through a catheter did not provide additional analgesia.[114] In a case-control study, patients undergoing cervical spinal fusion who received a pump providing a continuous subcutaneous infusion of 0.5% bupivacaine at 2 mL per hour for 72 hours experienced lower pain and required fewer narcotics than controls through postoperative day 4, were discharged sooner, and demonstrated improvements in time to the ambulation and discontinuation of PCA.[115] Another case-control study by the same investigators of patients undergoing lumbar fusion reported that patients who received subcutaneous infusion of 0.5% bupivacaine via a pump experienced lower pain scores for the first 5 postoperative days and required less opioid medication than did control patients.[116] Neither case-control study reported device-related adverse events.[115,116]

Extended Recovery After Surgery

Enhanced recovery after surgery (ERAS) is a multimodal approach to the care of surgical patients involving a multidisciplinary team of surgeons, anesthesiologists, ERAS program coordinators, and staff.[117] ERAS protocols involve preoperative, day of surgery, intraoperative, and postoperative components.[117] Preoperative elements include weight control, obstructive sleep apnea management, comorbidity guidance, and tobacco and alcohol cessation. Day of surgery aspects includes carbohydrate loading preoperatively (often with sports drinks), and preanesthesia medications, such as oral gabapentin or IV acetaminophen. Intraoperative components include IV ketamine, temperature management, and fluid management. Postoperative facets are early mobilization; early removal of urinary catheters; gum chewing to improve bowel function; and opioid alternatives, such as ketorolac, IV acetaminophen, gabapentin, and IV ketamine. Additional measures, such as absorbable skin sutures and avoidance of wound drains intraoperatively, use of dexmedetomidine, early extubation, and observation in a step-down unit are used in some ERAS protocols.[118,119] ERAS has been associated with reduced length of stay, total complications, and total costs after craniotomy.[120] A recent systematic review of ERAS in spine surgery reported shorter length of stay, decreased complication rates, and lower postoperative pain.[121] A systematic review of 9 studies, including 2 RCTs, on ERAS in cranial surgery demonstrated equivalent pain control between ERAS and conventional pathways.[122] However, the 2 RCTs reported improved pain control, shorter duration of pain, decreased length of stay, and improved Glasgow Outcome Scale and Modified Rankin Scale scores in the ERAS group relative to the non-ERAS group.[123,124] Neurosurgical patients tend to be satisfied with ERAS protocols.[125] Given the high variability in current ERAS protocols,[126] further research is required to determine if there is an optimal ERAS protocol for a given procedure.

Psychological Interventions

Cognitive-behavioral therapy (CBT) represents an important opportunity for decreasing pain following neurosurgery. CBT after cardiac surgery has been associated with improved pain and perceived control.[127] A systematic review of trials from multiple surgical fields revealed that psychological interventions involving CBT or a CBT-physiotherapy variant reduced the intensity of postsurgical pain and disability.[128] Similarly, an RCT involving CBT-based physical therapy for patients with chronic pain undergoing lumbar spine surgery found lower pain and disability at 6 months after surgery.[129] A recent meta-analysis of 7 studies with 531 patients undergoing lumbar spine surgery highlighted that CBT resulted in the greatest degree of improvement in quality of life and psychological outcomes and trended toward an improvement in pain.[130] Importantly, this strategy may be most effective in reducing pain when conducted twice weekly as originally intended.[130]

PATIENT-SPECIFIC CONSIDERATIONS FOR POSTOPERATIVE PAIN

The influence of patient-specific factors on postoperative pain control must also be considered. Significant predictors of patient-reported poor postoperative pain control include younger age, female sex, smoking, history of depression or anxiety symptoms, preoperative sleep difficulties, higher body mass index, presence of preoperative pain, and use of preoperative opioid analgesia.[131]

Studies have also examined the influence of patient demographics and baseline clinical status on postoperative pain following neurosurgery. Patients with preoperative pain experience more pain following craniotomy relative to those without, necessitating more intensive pain management.[4] Similarly, increased pain sensitivity and pain catastrophizing are both associated with greater postoperative pain intensity in patients undergoing lumbar spine surgery.[132] Preoperative depression is associated with increased cumulative opioid use, increased risk of chronic use, and decreased probability of opioid cessation after lumbar fusion.[133] Cannabis users report greater postoperative pain than nonusers.[134] The effects of age and gender are equivocal when considered alone.[135]

Clinical factors pertaining to neurosurgical procedures are also relevant to postoperative pain management. For example, patients who undergo infratentorial craniotomy experience greater pain than those who undergo supratentorial procedures, while patients with lumbar spine surgery have higher postoperative pain than those undergoing cervical procedures.[136] Frontal craniotomy patients may experience lower pain scores and consume less opioids than patients with posterior fossa craniotomy,[137] though another study found no differences in the severity of pain based on craniotomy site.[138]

Prediction rules have been created to try to identify which patients may experience poor postoperative pain relief based on demographic and clinical factors. One study identified younger age, female sex, preoperative daily use of opioid medications, higher preoperative neck or back pain intensity, higher Patient Health Questionnaire-9 depression score, surgery involving ≥ 2 motion segments, and fusion surgery as predictive of poor pain control.[139] Another study indicated that a prediction tool incorporating age, sex, race, insurance status, American Society of Anesthesiologists score, smoking status, diagnoses, prior surgery, prescription opioid use, asthma, and baseline PRO scores was useful in predicting pain reduction after lumbar fusion.[140]

Lastly, managing expectations is important. Patients who expect greater pain improvement following spine surgery experience a lower degree of pain improvement postoperatively.[141] Proper patient educational practices may be essential to calibrate expectations.[142,143] An understanding of these factors may enable neurosurgeons to tailor postoperative pain management strategies to the individual patient.

SUMMARY

Nonopioid management of postoperative pain is essential to improve postneurosurgical pain while reducing the postoperative use of opioids. An array of preoperative, intraoperative, and postoperative medication-based strategies exists. Multimodal, multidisciplinary approaches incorporating medical therapies, lifestyle modifications, clinical practices, and psychological interventions may provide optimal benefit. Consideration of patient-specific factors and the best-available evidence for interventions lays the foundation for the development of these approaches.

CLINICS CARE POINTS

- Preoperative medication options may be used to pre-emptively blunt postoperative pain.
- Pre-incision use of local anesthetic reduces postoperative opioid use.
- Ketorolac is a useful nonopioid medication for pain control that has not been shown to increase hemorrhage rate in patients undergoing craniotomy.
- ERAS protocols may lead to reduced postoperative pain and shorter length of stay.

DISCLOSURE

The authors have no conflicts of interest to disclose.

No part of this work has been previously published.

REFERENCES

1. De Benedittis S, Lorenzetti A, Migliore M, et al. Postoperative pain in neurosurgery: a pilot study in brain surgery. Neurosurgery 1996;38(3):466–70.
2. Mordhorst C, Latz B, Kerz T, et al. Prospective assessment of postoperative pain after craniotomy. J Neurosurg Anesthesiol 2010;22(3):202–6.
3. De Gray L, Matta B. Acute and chronic pain following craniotomy: a review. Anaesthesia 2005; 60(7):693–704.
4. Klimek M, Ubben JF, Ammann J, et al. Pain in neurosurgically treated patients: a prospective observational study. J Neurosurg 2006;104(3):350–9.
5. Kim YD, Park JH, Yang S-H, et al. Pain assessment in brain tumor patients after elective craniotomy. Brain Tumor Res Treat 2013;1(1):24–7.
6. Nair S, Rajshekhar V. Evaluation of pain following supratentorial craniotomy. Br J Neurosurg 2011; 25(1):100–3.
7. Turk DC, Okifuji A. Assessment of patients' reporting of pain: an integrated perspective. Lancet 1999;353(9166):1784–8.
8. Ossipov MH, Lai J, King T, et al. Antinociceptive and nociceptive actions of opioids. J Neurobiol 2004;61(1):126–48.
9. Benedetti F, Vighetti S, Amanzio M, et al. Dose-response relationship of opioids in nociceptive and neuropathic postoperative pain. Pain 1998; 74(2–3):205–11.
10. Yeung JC, Rudy TA. Sites of antinociceptive action of systemically injected morphine: involvement of supraspinal loci as revealed by intracerebroventricular injection of naloxone. J Pharmacol Exp Ther 1980;215(3):626–32.
11. Stanley B, Norman AF, Collins LJ, et al. Opioid prescribing in orthopaedic and neurosurgical specialties in a tertiary hospital: a retrospective audit of hospital discharge data. ANZ J Surg 2018; 88(11):1187–92.
12. Rautalin I, Kallio M, Korja M. In-hospital postoperative opioid use and its trends in neurosurgery between 2007 and 2018. Acta Neurochir 2021;1–10.
13. Yaeger KA, Rothrock RJ, Kopell BH. Commentary: neurosurgery and the ongoing american opioid crisis. Neurosurgery 2018;82(4):E79–90.
14. Khalid SI, Adogwa O, Lilly DT, et al. Opioid prescribing practices of neurosurgeons: analysis of medicare Part D. World Neurosurg 2018;112: e31–8.
15. Ricardo Buenaventura M, Rajive Adlaka M, Nalini Sehgal M. Opioid complications and side effects. Pain Physician 2008;11:S105–20.
16. Jordan B, Devi LA. Molecular mechanisms of opioid receptor signal transduction. Br J Anaesth 1998;81(1):12–9.
17. Trafton JA, Abbadie C, Marek K, et al. Postsynaptic signaling via the μ-opioid receptor: responses of dorsal horn neurons to exogenous opioids and noxious stimulation. J Neurosci 2000;20(23): 8578–84.
18. Borgland SL. Acute opioid receptor desensitization and tolerance: is there a link? Clin Exp Pharmacol Physiol 2001;28(3):147–54.
19. Gardell LR, Wang R, Burgess SE, et al. Sustained morphine exposure induces a spinal dynorphin-dependent enhancement of excitatory transmitter release from primary afferent fibers. J Neurosci 2002;22(15):6747–55.
20. Roberts G. A review of the efficacy and safety of opioid analgesics post-craniotomy. Nurs Crit Care 2004;9(6):277–83.
21. Yerneni K, Nichols N, Abecassis ZA, et al. Preoperative opioid use and clinical outcomes in spine

surgery: a systematic review. Neurosurgery 2020; 86(6):E490–507.

22. Volkow ND. Stigma and the toll of addiction. N Engl J Med 2020;382(14):1289–90.

23. McGinty EE, Barry CL. Stigma reduction to combat the addiction crisis—developing an evidence base. N Engl J Med 2020;382(14):1291–2.

24. Gourlay G, Wilson P, Glynn C. Pharmacodynamics and pharmacokinetics of methadone during the perioperative period. Anesthesiology 1982;57(6): 458–67.

25. Gottschalk A, Durieux ME, Nemergut EC. Intraoperative methadone improves postoperative pain control in patients undergoing complex spine surgery. Anesth Analg 2011;112(1):218–23.

26. Murphy GS, Szokol JW, Avram MJ, et al. Clinical effectiveness and safety of intraoperative methadone in patients undergoing posterior spinal fusion surgery: a randomized, double-blinded, controlled trial. Anesthesiology 2017;126(5):822–33.

27. Kukkar A, Bali A, Singh N, et al. Implications and mechanism of action of gabapentin in neuropathic pain. Arch Pharm Res 2013;36(3):237–51.

28. Tassone DM, Boyce E, Guyer J, et al. Pregabalin: a novel γ-aminobutyric acid analogue in the treatment of neuropathic pain, partial-onset seizures, and anxiety disorders. Clin Ther 2007;29(1):26–48.

29. Dahl JB, Mathiesen O, Møiniche S. 'Protective premedication': an option with gabapentin and related drugs? A review of gabapentin and pregabalin in the treatment of post-operative pain. Acta Anaesthesiol Scand 2004;48(9):1130–6.

30. Ho K-Y, Gan TJ, Habib AS. Gabapentin and postoperative pain–a systematic review of randomized controlled trials. Pain 2006;126(1–3):91–101.

31. Clarke H, Bonin RP, Orser BA, et al. The prevention of chronic postsurgical pain using gabapentin and pregabalin: a combined systematic review and meta-analysis. Anesth Analgesia 2012;115(2): 428–42.

32. Fabritius ML, Geisler A, Petersen PL, et al. Gabapentin in procedure-specific postoperative pain management–preplanned subgroup analyses from a systematic review with meta-analyses and trial sequential analyses. BMC anesthesiology 2017;17(1):1–20.

33. Fabritius M, Strøm C, Koyuncu S, et al. Benefit and harm of pregabalin in acute pain treatment: a systematic review with meta-analyses and trial sequential analyses. Br J Anaesth 2017;119(4):775–91.

34. Fabritius M, Geisler A, Petersen P, et al. Gabapentin for post-operative pain management–a systematic review with meta-analyses and trial sequential analyses. Acta Anaesthesiologica Scand 2016; 60(9):1188–208.

35. Türe H, Sayin M, Karlikaya G, et al. The analgesic effect of gabapentin as a prophylactic anticonvulsant drug on postcraniotomy pain: a prospective randomized study. Anesth Analgesia 2009;109(5):1625–31.

36. Zeng M, Dong J, Lin N, et al. Preoperative gabapentin administration improves acute postoperative analgesia in patients undergoing craniotomy: a randomized controlled trial. J Neurosurg Anesthesiol 2019;31(4):392–8.

37. Shimony N, Amit U, Minz B, et al. Perioperative pregabalin for reducing pain, analgesic consumption, and anxiety and enhancing sleep quality in elective neurosurgical patients: a prospective, randomized, double-blind, and controlled clinical study. J Neurosurg 2016;125(6):1513–22.

38. Yu L, Ran B, Li M, et al. Gabapentin and pregabalin in the management of postoperative pain after lumbar spinal surgery: a systematic review and meta-analysis. Spine 2013;38(22):1947–52.

39. Urban MK, Labib KM, Reid SC, et al. Pregabalin did not improve pain management after spinal fusions. HSS Journal® 2018;14(1):41–6.

40. Ventham NT, O'Neill S, Johns N, et al. Evaluation of novel local anesthetic wound infiltration techniques for postoperative pain following colorectal resection surgery: a meta-analysis. Dis Colon Rectum 2014;57(2):237–50.

41. Adesope O, Ituk U, Habib AS. Local anaesthetic wound infiltration for postcaesarean section analgesia: a systematic review and meta-analysis. Eur J Anaesthesiol| 2016;33(10):731–42.

42. Song J, Li L, Yu P, et al. Preemptive scalp infiltration with 0.5% ropivacaine and 1% lidocaine reduces postoperative pain after craniotomy. Acta neurochirurgica 2015;157(6):993–8.

43. Biswas BK, Bithal PK. Preincision 0.25% bupivacaine scalp infiltration and postcraniotomy pain a randomized double-blind, placebo-controlled study. J Neurosurg Anesthesiology 2003;15(3): 234–9.

44. Torun F, Mordeniz C, Baysal Z, et al. Intraoperative perineural infiltration of lidocaine for acute postlaminectomy pain: preemptive analgesia in spinal surgery. Clin Spine Surg 2010;23(1):43–6.

45. Perera AP, Chari A, Kostusiak M, et al. Intramuscular local anesthetic infiltration at closure for postoperative analgesia in lumbar spine surgery: a systematic review and meta-analysis. Spine 2017; 42(14):1088–95.

46. Tedavisinde LLSPA, İnfiltrasyonu PYY, ve Levobupivakain'in B. Preemptive wound infiltration in lumbar laminectomy for postoperative pain: comparison of bupivacaine and levobupivacaine. Turkish Neurosurg 2014;24(1):48–53.

47. Kjaergaard M, Møiniche S, Olsen K. Wound infiltration with local anesthetics for post-operative pain relief in lumbar spine surgery: a systematic review. Acta Anaesthesiologica Scand 2012;56(3):282–90.

48. Yörükoglu D, Ates Y, Temiz H, et al. Comparison of low-dose intrathecal and epidural morphine and bupivacaine infiltration for postoperative pain control after surgery for lumbar disc disease. J Neurosurg Anesthesiology 2005;17(3):129–33.

49. Abdel Hay J, Kobaiter-Maarrawi S, Tabet P, et al. Bupivacaine field block with clonidine for postoperative pain control in posterior spine approaches: a randomized double-blind trial. Neurosurgery 2018; 82(6):790–8.

50. Galvin IM, Levy R, Day AG, et al. Pharmacological interventions for the prevention of acute postoperative pain in adults following brain surgery. Cochrane Database Syst Rev 2019;2019(11): CD011931.

51. Law-Koune J-D, Szekely B, Fermanian C, et al. Scalp infiltration with bupivacaine plus epinephrine or plain ropivacaine reduces postoperative pain after supratentorial craniotomy. J Neurosurg Anesthesiology 2005;17(3):139–43.

52. Akcil EF, Dilmen OK, Vehid H, et al. Which one is more effective for analgesia in infratentorial craniotomy? The scalp block or local anesthetic infiltration. Clin Neurol Neurosurg 2017;154:98–103.

53. Kassem AA, Youssef A, Ahmed N, et al. Scalp block versus subcutaneous infiltration for stereotactic brain biopsy: a randomized controlled trial. Res Opin Anesth Intensive Care 2019;6(1):134.

54. Chaki T, Sugino S, Janicki PK, et al. Efficacy and safety of a lidocaine and ropivacaine mixture for scalp nerve block and local infiltration anesthesia in patients undergoing awake craniotomy. J Neurosurg Anesthesiology 2016;28(1):1–5.

55. Guilfoyle MR, Helmy A, Duane D, et al. Regional scalp block for postcraniotomy analgesia: a systematic review and meta-analysis. Anesth Analgesia 2013;116(5):1093–102.

56. Krauss P, Marahori NA, Oertel MF, et al. Better hemodynamics and less antihypertensive medication: comparison of scalp block and local infiltration anesthesia for skull-pin placement in awake deep brain stimulation surgery. World Neurosurg 2018;120:e991–9.

57. Rigamonti A, Garavaglia MM, Ma K, et al. Effect of bilateral scalp nerve blocks on postoperative pain and discharge times in patients undergoing supratentorial craniotomy and general anesthesia: a randomized-controlled trial. Can J Anesth 2020; 67(4):452–61.

58. Bhakta P, Dash H. Bilateral scalp blocks help reduce postoperative pain and opioid requirement, but the impact cannot be so huge. Can J Anesth 2020;67(9):1294–5.

59. Glasser RS, Knego RS, Delashaw JB, et al. The perioperative use of corticosteroids and bupivacaine in the management of lumbar disc disease. J Neurosurg 1993;78(3):383–7.

60. Mirzai H, Tekin I, Alincak H. Perioperative use of corticosteroid and bupivacaine combination in lumbar disc surgery: a randomized controlled trial. Spine 2002;27(4):343–6.

61. Jirarattanaphochai K, Jung S, Thienthong S, et al. Peridural methylprednisolone and wound infiltration with bupivacaine for postoperative pain control after posterior lumbar spine surgery: a randomized double-blinded placebo-controlled trial. Spine 2007;32(6):609–16.

62. Bahari S, El-Dahab M, Cleary M, et al. Efficacy of triamcinolone acetonide and bupivacaine for pain after lumbar discectomy. Eur Spine J 2010;19(7): 1099–103.

63. Akinduro OO, Miller BA, Haussen DC, et al. Complications of intraoperative epidural steroid use in lumbar discectomy: a systematic review and meta-analysis. Neurosurg Focus 2015;39(4):E12.

64. Wilson-Smith A, Chang N, Lu VM, et al. Epidural steroids at closure after microdiscectomy/laminectomy for reduction of postoperative analgesia: systematic review and meta-analysis. World Neurosurg 2018;110:e212–21.

65. Machado FC, Vieira JE, Flávia A, et al. Intraoperative methadone reduces pain and opioid consumption in acute postoperative pain: a systematic review and meta-analysis. Anesth Analgesia 2019;129(6):1723–32.

66. D'Souza RS, Gurrieri C, Johnson RL, et al. Intraoperative methadone administration and postoperative pain control: a systematic review and meta-analysis. Pain 2020;161(2):237–43.

67. Dunn LK, Yerra S, Fang S, et al. Safety profile of intraoperative methadone for analgesia after major spine surgery: an observational study of 1,478 patients. J Opioid Manag 2018;14(2):83.

68. Brinck EC, Tiippana E, Heesen M, et al. Perioperative intravenous ketamine for acute postoperative pain in adults. Cochrane Database Syst Rev 2018;12(12):CD012033.

69. Loftus RW, Yeager MP, Clark JA, et al. Intraoperative ketamine reduces perioperative opiate consumption in opiate-dependent patients with chronic back pain undergoing back surgery. J Am Soc Anesthesiologists 2010;113(3):639–46.

70. Nielsen RV, Fomsgaard JS, Siegel H, et al. Intraoperative ketamine reduces immediate postoperative opioid consumption after spinal fusion surgery in chronic pain patients with opioid dependency: a randomized, blinded trial. Pain 2017; 158(3):463–70.

71. Boenigk K, Echevarria GC, Nisimov E, et al. Low-dose ketamine infusion reduces postoperative hydromorphone requirements in opioid-tolerant patients following spinal fusion: a randomised controlled trial. Eur J Anaesthesiol 2019;36(1): 8–15.

72. Wang X, Ding X, Tong Y, et al. Ketamine does not increase intracranial pressure compared with opioids: meta-analysis of randomized controlled trials. J Anesth 2014;28(6):821–7.

73. Remy C, Marret E, Bonnet F. Effects of acetaminophen on morphine side-effects and consumption after major surgery: meta-analysis of randomized controlled trials. Br J Anaesth 2005;94(4):505–13.

74. Sivakumar W, Jensen M, Martinez J, et al. Intravenous acetaminophen for postoperative supratentorial craniotomy pain: a prospective, randomized, double-blinded, placebo-controlled trial. J Neurosurg 2018;130(3):766-722.

75. Greenberg S, Murphy GS, Avram MJ, et al. Postoperative intravenous acetaminophen for craniotomy patients: a randomized controlled trial. World Neurosurg 2018;109:e554–62.

76. Artime C, Aijazi H, Zhang H, et al. Scheduled intravenous acetaminophen improves patient satisfaction with postcraniotomy pain management: A prospective, randomized, placebo-controlled, double-blind study. J Neurosurg Anesthesiology 2018; 30(3):231.

77. Ghaffarpasand F, Dadgostar E, Ilami G, et al. Intravenous acetaminophen (paracetamol) for postcraniotomy pain: systematic review and meta-analysis of randomized controlled trials. World Neurosurg 2020;134:569–76.

78. Mörwald EE, Poeran J, Zubizarreta N, et al. Intravenous acetaminophen does not reduce inpatient opioid prescription or opioid-related adverse events among patients undergoing spine surgery. Anesth Analgesia 2018;127(5):1221–8.

79. Hiller A, Helenius I, Nurmi E, et al. Acetaminophen improves analgesia but does not reduce opioid requirement after major spine surgery in children and adolescents. Spine 2012;37(20):E1225–31.

80. Hansen RN, Pham AT, Böing EA, et al. Comparative analysis of length of stay, hospitalization costs, opioid use, and discharge status among spine surgery patients with postoperative pain management including intravenous versus oral acetaminophen. Curr Med Res Opin 2017;33(5):943–8.

81. Forrest J, Camu F, Greer I, et al. Ketorolac, diclofenac, and ketoprofen are equally safe for pain relief after major surgery. Br J Anaesth 2002;88(2):227–33.

82. Le Roux PD, Samudrala S. Postoperative pain after lumbar disc surgery: a comparison between parenteral ketorolac and narcotics. Acta Neurochirurgica 1999;141(3):261–7.

83. Kim H-S, Choi K-H, Han T-H. IV ketorolac combined with morphine PCA in postoperative pain control after lumbar disc surgery. Korean J Pain 2000;13(2): 218–23.

84. Reuben SS, Connelly NR, Steinberg R. Ketorolac as an adjunct to patient-controlled morphine in postoperative spine surgery patients. Reg Anesth Pain Med 1997;22(4):343–6.

85. Reuben SS, Connelly NR, Lurie S, et al. Dose-response of ketorolac as an adjunct to patient-controlled analgesia morphine in patients after spinal fusion surgery. Anesth Analgesia 1998;87(1): 98–102.

86. Pace V, Gul A, Prakash V, et al. Wound Infiltration with Levobupivacaine, Ketorolac, and Adrenaline for Postoperative Pain Control after Spinal Fusion Surgery. Asian Spine J 2021;15(4):539.

87. Mack PF, Hass D, Lavyne MH, et al. Postoperative narcotic requirement after microscopic lumbar discectomy is not affected by intraoperative ketorolac or bupivacaine. Spine 2001;26(6):658–61.

88. Richardson MD, Palmeri NO, Williams SA, et al. Routine perioperative ketorolac administration is not associated with hemorrhage in pediatric neurosurgery patients. J Neurosurg Pediatr 2016;17(1): 107–15.

89. Magni G, La Rosa I, Melillo G, et al. Intracranial hemorrhage requiring surgery in neurosurgical patients given ketorolac: a case-control study within a cohort (2001–2010). Anesth Analgesia 2013; 116(2):443–7.

90. Park S-Y, Moon S-H, Park M-S, et al. The effects of ketorolac injected via patient controlled analgesia postoperatively on spinal fusion. Yonsei Med J 2005;46(2):245–51.

91. Sucato DJ, Lovejoy JF, Agrawal S, et al. Postoperative ketorolac does not predispose to pseudoarthrosis following posterior spinal fusion and instrumentation for adolescent idiopathic scoliosis. Spine 2008;33(10):1119–24.

92. Pradhan BB, Tatsumi RL, Gallina J, et al. Ketorolac and spinal fusion: does the perioperative use of ketorolac really inhibit spinal fusion? Spine 2008; 33(19):2079–82.

93. Li Q, Zhang Z, Cai Z. High-dose ketorolac affects adult spinal fusion: a meta-analysis of the effect of perioperative nonsteroidal anti-inflammatory drugs on spinal fusion. Spine 2011;36(7):E461–8.

94. Chahar P, Cummings KC III. Liposomal bupivacaine: a review of a new bupivacaine formulation. J Pain Res 2012;5:257.

95. Kim J, Burke SM, Kryzanski JT, et al. The role of liposomal bupivacaine in reduction of postoperative pain after transforaminal lumbar interbody fusion: a clinical study. World Neurosurg 2016;91:460–7.

96. Grieff AN, Ghobrial GM, Jallo J. Use of liposomal bupivacaine in the postoperative management of posterior spinal decompression. J Neurosurg Spine 2016;25(1):88–93.

97. Katsevman GA, Allison AA, Fang W, et al. Retrospective Assessment of the Use of Liposomal Bupivacaine in Lumbar Fusions in Immediate

Postoperative Hospital Care. World Neurosurg 2020;141:e820–8.

98. Lu VM, Daniels DJ, Haile DT, et al. Effects of intraoperative liposomal bupivacaine on pain control and opioid use after pediatric Chiari I malformation surgery: an initial experience. J Neurosurg Pediatr 2020;27(1):9–15.

99. Mantz J, Josserand J, Hamada S. Dexmedetomidine: new insights. Eur J Anaesthesiology 2011; 28(1):3–6.

100. Blaudszun G, Lysakowski C, Elia N, et al. Effect of perioperative systemic α2 agonists on postoperative morphine consumption and pain intensity: systematic review and meta-analysis of randomized controlled trials. J Am Soc Anesthesiologists 2012;116(6):1312–22.

101. Schnabel A, Meyer-Frießem C, Reichl S, et al. Is intraoperative dexmedetomidine a new option for postoperative pain treatment? A meta-analysis of randomized controlled trials. Pain 2013;154(7): 1140–9.

102. Bellon M, Le Bot A, Michelet D, et al. Efficacy of intraoperative dexmedetomidine compared with placebo for postoperative pain management: a meta-analysis of published studies. Pain Ther 2016;5(1): 63–80.

103. Le Bot A, Michelet D, Hilly J, et al. Efficacy of intraoperative dexmedetomidine compared with placebo for surgery in adults: a meta-analysis of published studies. Minerva Anestesiol 2015; 81(10):1105–17.

104. Peng K, Jin X-H, Liu S-L, et al. Effect of intraoperative dexmedetomidine on post-craniotomy pain. Clin Ther 2015;37(5):1114–21.e1.

105. Su S, Ren C, Zhang H, et al. The opioid-sparing effect of perioperative dexmedetomidine plus sufentanil infusion during neurosurgery: a retrospective study. Front Pharmacol 2016;7:407.

106. Liu Y, Liang F, Liu X, et al. Dexmedetomidine reduces perioperative opioid consumption and postoperative pain intensity in neurosurgery: a meta-analysis. J Neurosurg Anesthesiology 2018;30(2): 146–55.

107. Wang L, Shen J, Ge L, et al. Dexmedetomidine for craniotomy under general anesthesia: a systematic review and meta-analysis of randomized clinical trials. J Clin Anesth 2019;54:114–25.

108. Salem R, Darweesh E, Wanis M, et al. Evaluation of the effects of intrathecal bupivacaine-dexmedetomidine for lumbar spine fusion: a double blinded randomized controlled study. Eur Rev Med Pharmacol Sci 2015;19(23):4542–8.

109. Bojaxhi E, Louie C, ReFaey K, et al. Reduced pain and opioid use in the early postoperative period in patients undergoing a frontotemporal craniotomy under regional vs general anesthesia. World Neurosurg 2021;150:e31–7.

110. Liu SS, Richman JM, Thirlby RC, et al. Efficacy of continuous wound catheters delivering local anesthetic for postoperative analgesia: a quantitative and qualitative systematic review of randomized controlled trials. J Am Coll Surg 2006;203(6): 914–32.

111. Raines S, Hedlund C, Franzon M, et al. Ropivacaine for continuous wound infusion for postoperative pain management: a systematic review and meta-analysis of randomized controlled trials. Eur Surg Res 2014;53(1–4):43–60.

112. Mekawy NM, Badawy SS, Sakr SA. Role of postoperative continuous subfascial bupivacaine infusion after posterior cervical laminectomy: Randomized control study. Egypt J Anaesth 2012;28(1):83–8.

113. Lee S-M, Yun D-J, Lee S-H, et al. Continuous wound infiltration of ropivacaine for reducing of postoperative pain after anterior lumbar fusion surgery: a clinical retrospective comparative study. Korean J Pain 2021;34(2):193.

114. Grèze J, Vighetti A, Incagnoli P, et al. Does continuous wound infiltration enhance baseline intravenous multimodal analgesia after posterior spinal fusion surgery? A randomized, double-blinded, placebo-controlled study. Eur Spine J 2017;26(3): 832–9.

115. Elder JB, Hoh DJ, Liu CY, et al. Postoperative continuous paravertebral anesthetic infusion for pain control in posterior cervical spine surgery: a case-control study. Oper Neurosurg 2010; 66(suppl_1). ons-99–ons-107.

116. Elder JB, Hoh DJ, Wang MY. Postoperative continuous paravertebral anesthetic infusion for pain control in lumbar spinal fusion surgery. Spine 2008;33(2):210–8.

117. Ljungqvist O, Scott M, Fearon KC. Enhanced recovery after surgery: a review. JAMA Surg 2017; 152(3):292–8.

118. Stumpo V, Staartjes VE, Quddusi A, et al. Enhanced Recovery After Surgery strategies for elective craniotomy: a systematic review. J Neurosurg 2021;1(aop):1–25.

119. Kaye AD, Chernobylsky DJ, Thakur P, et al. Dexmedetomidine in enhanced recovery after surgery (ERAS) protocols for postoperative pain. Curr Pain Headache Rep 2020;24(5):1–13.

120. Lau CS, Chamberlain RS. Enhanced recovery after surgery programs improve patient outcomes and recovery: a meta-analysis. World J Surg 2017; 41(4):899–913.

121. Pennington Z, Cottrill E, Lubelski D, et al. Systematic review and meta-analysis of the clinical utility of Enhanced Recovery After Surgery pathways in adult spine surgery. J Neurosurg Spine 2020; 34(2):325–47.

122. Peters EJ, Robinson M, Serletis D. Systematic Review of Enhanced Recovery After Surgery in

Patients Undergoing Cranial Surgery. World Neurosurg 2021;S1878-8750(21):01687-9.

123. Wang Y, Liu B, Zhao T, et al. Safety and efficacy of a novel neurosurgical enhanced recovery after surgery protocol for elective craniotomy: a prospective randomized controlled trial. J Neurosurg 2018;130(5):1680-91.

124. Han H, Guo S, Jiang H, et al. Feasibility and efficacy of enhanced recovery after surgery protocol in Chinese elderly patients with intracranial aneurysm. Clin Interventions Aging 2019;14:203.

125. Liu B, Liu S, Wang Y, et al. Neurosurgical enhanced recovery after surgery (ERAS) programme for elective craniotomies: are patients satisfied with their experiences? A quantitative and qualitative analysis. BMJ open 2019;9(11):e028706.

126. Dietz N, Sharma M, Adams S, et al. Enhanced recovery after surgery (ERAS) for spine surgery: a systematic review. World Neurosurg 2019;130:415-26.

127. Doering LV, McGuire A, Eastwood J-A, et al. Cognitive behavioral therapy for depression improves pain and perceived control in cardiac surgery patients. Eur J Cardiovasc Nurs 2016;15(6):417-24.

128. Nicholls JL, Azam MA, Burns LC, et al. Psychological treatments for the management of postsurgical pain: a systematic review of randomized controlled trials. Patient Relat Outcome Measures 2018;9:49.

129. Archer KR, Devin CJ, Vanston SW, et al. Cognitive-behavioral-based physical therapy for patients with chronic pain undergoing lumbar spine surgery: a randomized controlled trial. J Pain 2016;17(1):76-89.

130. Parrish JM, Jenkins NW, Parrish MS, et al. The influence of cognitive behavioral therapy on lumbar spine surgery outcomes: a systematic review and meta-analysis. Eur Spine J 2021;1-15.

131. Yang MM, Hartley RL, Leung AA, et al. Preoperative predictors of poor acute postoperative pain control: a systematic review and meta-analysis. BMJ Open 2019;9(4):e025091.

132. Coronado RA, George SZ, Devin CJ, et al. Pain sensitivity and pain catastrophizing are associated with persistent pain and disability after lumbar spine surgery. Arch Phys Med Rehabil 2015;96(10):1763-70.

133. O'Connell C, Azad TD, Mittal V, et al. Preoperative depression, lumbar fusion, and opioid use: an assessment of postoperative prescription, quality, and economic outcomes. Neurosurg Focus 2018;44(1):E5.

134. Dupriest K, Rogers K, Thakur B, et al. Postoperative pain management is influenced by previous cannabis use in neurosurgical patients. J Neurosci Nurs 2021;53(2):87-91.

135. Chowdhury T, Garg R, Sheshadri V, et al. Perioperative factors contributing the post-craniotomy pain: a synthesis of concepts. Front Med 2017;4:23.

136. Dhandapani M, Dhandapani S, Agarwal M, et al. Pain perception following different neurosurgical procedures: a quantitative prospective study. Contemp Nurse 2016;52(4):477-85.

137. Thibault M, Girard F, Chouinard P, et al. Craniotomy site influences postoperative pain following neurosurgical procedures: a retrospective study. Can J Anesth 2007;54(7):544-8.

138. Irefin SA, Schubert A, Bloomfield EL, et al. The effect of craniotomy location on postoperative pain and nausea. J Anesth 2003;17(4):227-31.

139. Yang MM, Riva-Cambrin J, Cunningham J, et al. Development and validation of a clinical prediction score for poor postoperative pain control following elective spine surgery: Presented at the 2020 AANS/CNS Joint Section on Disorders of the Spine and Peripheral Nerves. J Neurosurg Spine 2020;34(1):3-12.

140. Khor S, Lavallee D, Cizik AM, et al. Development and validation of a prediction model for pain and functional outcomes after lumbar spine surgery. JAMA Surg 2018;153(7):634-42.

141. Mancuso CA, Reid MC, Duculan R, et al. Improvement in pain after lumbar spine surgery: the role of preoperative expectations of pain relief. Clin J Pain 2017;33(2):93.

142. Shlobin NA, Clark JR, Hoffman SC, et al. Patient education in neurosurgery: part 1 of a systematic review. World Neurosurg 2021;147:190-201.e1.

143. Shlobin NA, Clark JR, Hoffman SC, et al. Patient education in neurosurgery: part 2 of a systematic review. World Neurosurg 2021;147:190-201.e1.

Mindfulness Meditation in the Treatment of Chronic Pain

Michael G. Brandel, MD, MAS[a], Christine Lin, BA[a], Devon Hennel, MS[b],
Olga Khazen, MS[b], Julie G. Pilitsis, MD, PhD[c], Sharona Ben-Haim, MD[a],*

KEYWORDS

• Chronic pain • Mindfulness • Meditation • Functional neuroimaging • Neural network

KEY POINTS

• Chronic pain has a significant impact on quality of life, medical expenses, and lost productivity.
• Mindfulness meditation has proven to be efficacious in reducing pain in patients with chronic pain.
• Evidence from functional neuroimaging studies may provide insight into the mechanism by which mindfulness-based interventions treat chronic pain.

PAIN

Pain is a distressing sensation and emotional experience which may be linked to actual or potential tissue damage.[1] Chronic pain may be a result of peripheral tissue damage, including inflammation, alone or in combination with pathologic adaptations of the nervous system.[2] While the neural mechanisms of chronic pain are incompletely understood, multiple animal studies describe activity-dependent changes in gene expression in the spinal cord and cerebral cortex. Therefore, treatments that work locally or via a single signaling pathway are unsurprisingly limited in their efficacy for chronic pain.[3]

Nociceptive sensory afferents travel from the periphery to the dorsal horn of the spinal cord via Aδ fibers (small, myelinated, and relatively fast thermal and mechanical nociceptors) and C-fibers (small, unmyelinated, slow, and polymodal). Nociceptive information then ascends contralaterally within the spinothalamic pathway to the periaqueductal (PAG) gray matter, thalamus, and primary/secondary somatosensory cortices. This information is then processed by the insula and interpreted by the dorsal anterior cingulate cortex (dACC), prefrontal cortex (PFC), and posterior parietal cortex in a complex interplay often dubbed the "Pain Matrix."[4]

Pain is tridimensional, consisting of sensory, affective, and emotional components. Two pathways for pain exist. The lateral pathway is related to the sensory component of pain and involves the thalamus and somatosensory cortices while the medial pathway encompasses the affective and emotional components.[5,6] Previous fMRI studies in chronic pain patients have demonstrated altered functional connections between sensory and affective regions, suggesting that the lateral pathway works in parallel with the medial pathway.[7,8] Due to this dynamic relationship of the lateral and medial pathways, it is suggested that changes in neural correlates may be associated with how pain is processed during mindfulness intervention.

MINDFULNESS

Mindfulness is a process involving awareness of the present moment experience.[9] Two major forms of mindfulness-based practice are Shamatha (focused attention) and Vipassana (open monitoring/choiceless awareness).[10,11] In the practice of focused attention, attention is placed on a

a Department of Neurosurgery, University of California, 200 W. Arbor Drive #8893, USA; b Department of Neuroscience & Experimental Therapeutics, Albany Medical College, Albany, NY, USA; c Department of Biomedical Research, Florida Atlantic University, Boca Raton, Florida, USA
* Corresponding author.
E-mail address: sbenhaim@health.ucsd.edu

Neurosurg Clin N Am 33 (2022) 275–279
https://doi.org/10.1016/j.nec.2022.02.005
1042-3680/22/© 2022 Elsevier Inc. All rights reserved.

dynamic, automatic stimulus such as breathing. With increased experience and expertise in Shamatha, there is natural evolution to Vipassana, which involves meta-awareness of sensory, affective, or cognitive events, which can then be deliberately "let go" without reflexively engaging with the event.[12,13] While there has been a scholarly focus on mindfulness in the context of pain management over the past few decades, it has been an essential component of Buddhist teachings for millenia.[14] Recent studies have shown positive outcomes following the implementation of mindfulness programs to treat chronic pain patients. Specifically, studies noted reductions in functional limitations, present moment pain, negative body image, mood changes, anxiety, and depression.[15–17] However, the programs used in these studies were lengthy and intensive lasting between 3 weeks and 3 months.[18] Implementation of such programs may be hindered by a low rate of adherence to programs involving lifestyle changes and noncompliance results in poor outcomes and recurrent pain.[19–21] Thus, the use of brief mindfulness-based intervention (bMBI) should be explored as an alternative treatment of chronic pain.

Neuroimaging

EEG

Changes in EEG have been useful in comparing brain activity before mindfulness and after mindfulness. Beta and gamma powers are associated with higher processing, anxiety, and critical thinking, whereas alpha power is associated with a more positive and relaxed mental state.[22,23] In healthy controls, EEG has shown an increase in delta activity, reduction in theta and alpha activity in the left frontotemporal region, and an increase in beta activity in the left temporal region following mindfulness.[24] Further, global alpha activity has been previously found to increase during meditation, and to be higher at baseline in experienced meditators.[25] In a study of individuals with chronic pain undergoing meditation training, Jensen and colleagues found that lower baseline alpha power correlated with higher pain reductions after meditative intervention.[26] An RCT evaluating a mindfulness intervention in women undergoing breast biopsy identified higher beta current source density (CSD) in the insula compared with controls and increases in theta CSD in the medial prefrontal cortex (MPFC), insula, and ACC, areas known to be associated with self-awareness.[27] Meditation was associated with reduced anxiety during breast biopsy but did not impact pain.

Brown and Jones investigated the impact of long-term mindfulness practice on event-related potentials (ERPs) from painful laser stimuli compared with control subjects without mediation experience.[28] Experienced meditators had lower pain unpleasantness ratings, which were thought to represent a reduced affective response to pain. Additionally, meditation was associated with smaller anticipation-evoked potentials to noxious stimuli in right inferior parietal cortex and mid-cingulate cortex (MCC). Lower unpleasantness ratings were directly related to lower MCC activation in meditators but not controls. Meditators had increased the activation of the dACC and ventromedial PFC compared with controls; activation in these regions was positively associated with pain unpleasantness in controls and negatively in meditators, suggesting that meditation experience may have remodeled the processing of nociceptive information in a sustained fashion.

Current research has called attention to the benefits of increased awareness, being present in the moment, and reducing attachment to different emotions or states of being. Brown and colleagues implemented an 8-week mindfulness intervention for patients with chronic pain and reported significant deactivations within the dorsolateral prefrontal cortex (DLPFC) and secondary somatosensory cortices (S2) during the anticipatory phase of pain.[29] Patients who did not undergo mindfulness intervention had higher activation in the DLPFC and S2 during the anticipatory phase.[29] Zeidan and colleagues reported similar results showing differing activation of DLPFC and S2 due to mindfulness thus concluding the intervention was associated with the modulation of pain.[30]

MR imaging

In studies comparing pain-evoked fMRI activity during meditation and at rest between expert and novice meditators, greater activation of primary somatosensory cortices was demonstrated in experienced meditators while there was reduced activation in novice meditators. Additionally, in novice meditators, decreased activation of the thalamus and PAG and increased activation of the insula and S2 were seen among healthy participants.[30,31] Gard and colleagues found that mindfulness practitioners had increased activation in the rostral ACC while anticipating pain in a state of mindfulness, but not in controls.[32] The receipt of painful stimuli in a state of mindfulness was associated with decreased activation of the lateral PFCs and increased activation in the posterior insula/secondary somatosensory cortex (S2). Zeidan and colleagues used arterial spin labeling (ASL) fMRI to assess the impact of mindfulness meditation in the setting of a noxious stimulus on cerebral blood flow and various pain measurements.[30,33] Meditation reduced activation in the contralateral primary somatosensory cortex. Furthermore, meditation reduced pain via several mechanisms, including increased activation in the rACC, right anterior insula, and OFC. These findings were also consistent with studies comparing mindfulness meditation to sham mindfulness interventions and analyzing the pain reduction mechanisms of Zen meditation.[31,34] Zeidan and colleagues further described the neuroanatomic-specific mechanisms by which mindfulness meditation modulates pain response.[31] Activation of the right anterior insula probably fine-tuned sensory evaluations in a context-dependent manner.[35] ACC activation likely mediated attentional shifts between endogenous and exogenous stimuli.[36] Activation of the OFC may represent adjustment of the contextual evaluation of nociceptive sensory events by unique reappraisal processes.[37,38]

Clinical Effectiveness

The efficacy of mindfulness-based interventions (MBIs) has been studied across a range of pain-related conditions, with the 8-week mindfulness-based stress reduction (MBSR) program being the most studied intervention.[39] Current research is focused on understanding the mechanism of MBI, how much MBI training is needed for various conditions, and how to effectively quantify the effects.[9] A meta-analysis by Hilton and colleagues analyzed the results of over 3000 total patients enrolled in 30 RCTs, finding that mindfulness meditation was associated with improved chronic pain symptoms compared with standard treatment, passive controls, and education/support groups.[18] However, the effect size was small and there was substantial heterogeneity in results and quality among the studies.

A few landmark studies provide support for the use of MBIs in chronic pain treatment. In 1982, Kabat-Zinn demonstrated that a 10-week MBSR program resulted in sustained pain reduction and affect improvement among 51 patients with chronic pain, including when patients were re-evaluated several years later.[15] A single-blind RCT of 282 adults greater than age 65 with CLBP comparing an 8-week MBSR to a health education program showed improved pain ratings in the MBSR group, as well as short-term functional status, although this was not sustained at 6 months follow-up.[40] Numerous studies demonstrated that mindfulness interventions improved affective pain (more so than sensory pain),[32,33,41] or affective components that relate to the experience of pain

such as depression, stress, or pain acceptance.[42–45] The effect of mindfulness on pain has also been demonstrated in models of experimentally induced pain. In a randomized study of 78 pain-free participants, Case and colleagues analyzed the pain ratings in response to meditation or rest (control group) during a noxious stimulus with the concurrent administration of naloxone or placebo.[46] They found that mindfulness significantly lowered pain and that this effect persisted even among subjects with low expectations for pain relief. Zeidan and colleagues randomized 75 healthy participants to mindfulness meditation, placebo, sham mindfulness meditation, or control before receiving a noxious thermal stimulus.[31] Mindfulness-meditation-related pain relief was found to be mechanistically distinct from placebo or sham mindfulness meditation conditions, and reduced pain intensity and unpleasantness ratings beyond the analgesic effects of these other interventions.

Overall, MBI has been found to be effective in a range of disorders and has been shown to improve awareness, calmness, and sense of well-being.[47] In a clinical context, it is important to be aware that MBI is aimed to reduce suffering, not necessarily treat an illness. Like any treatment, this intervention may not work for everyone so careful selection of candidates is important for optimal pain relief and prevention of recurrent pain.

FUTURE DIRECTIONS

Recent research has highlighted the potential of mindfulness meditation to mitigate pain in patients with chronic pain. Future studies should analyze the effect of mindfulness-based interventions on spatiotemporal dynamics, brain activation patterns, and connectivity in chronic pain patients using multiple modalities, including fMRI and EEG. In light of the limitations of self-reported outcomes, an investigation of biomarkers to evaluate the effect of interventions on chronic pain is needed. Additionally, a better understanding of how mindfulness-based interventions alter functionality and connectivity may improve their efficacy and solidify their role in the cognitive and behavioral treatments of chronic pain. The ease and brevity of mindfulness meditation make it suitable for incorporation into patients' daily routines and serve as a promising option for mitigating pain and reducing disability. Mindfulness is a difficult task and is not feasible for every individual due to personal, interpersonal, and contextual factors.[47] Thus, additional research on individual differences between patients and the efficacy of MBI is imperative to ensure that patients are appropriately selected for this intervention.

DISCLOSURE

The authors have nothing to disclose.

REFERENCES

1. Yam MF, Loh YC, Tan CS, et al. General pathways of pain sensation and the major neurotransmitters involved in pain regulation. Int J Mol Sci 2018; 19(8):2164.
2. Descalzi G, Ikegami D, Ushijima T, et al. Epigenetic mechanisms of chronic pain. Trends Neurosci 2015; 38(4):237–46.
3. Coghill RC, Talbot JD, Evans AC, et al. Distributed processing of pain and vibration by the human brain. J Neurosci 1994;14(7):4095–108.
4. Salomons TV, Iannetti GD, Liang M, et al. The "pain matrix" in pain-free individuals. JAMA Neurol 2016; 73(6):755–6.
5. Bushnell MC, Ceko M, Low LA. Cognitive and emotional control of pain and its disruption in chronic pain. Nat Rev Neurosci 2013;14(7):502–11.
6. Price DD. Psychological and neural mechanisms of the affective dimension of pain. Science 2000; 288(5472):1769–72.
7. Malinen S, Vartiainen N, Hlushchuk Y, et al. Aberrant temporal and spatial brain activity during rest in patients with chronic pain. Proc Natl Acad Sci U S A 2010;107(14):6493–7.
8. Cauda F, D'Agata F, Sacco K, et al. Altered resting state attentional networks in diabetic neuropathic pain. J Neurol Neurosurg Psychiatr 2010;81(7):806–11.
9. Creswell JD. Mindfulness interventions. Annu Rev Psychol 2017;68:491–516.
10. Lutz A, Slagter HA, Dunne JD, et al. Attention regulation and monitoring in meditation. Trends Cogn Sci 2008;12(4):163–9.
11. Wallace BA. The attention revolution: unlocking the power of the focused mind. Manhattan, New York City: Simon and Schuster; 2006.
12. Zeidan F, Baumgartner JN, Coghill RC. The neural mechanisms of mindfulness-based pain relief: a functional magnetic resonance imaging-based review and primer. Pain Rep 2019;4(4):e759.
13. Schooler JW, Smallwood J, Christoff K, et al. Meta-awareness, perceptual decoupling and the wandering mind. Trends Cogn Sci 2011;15(7):319–26.
14. Analayo B. Sattipatthana: the direct path to realization. Birmingham, United Kingdom: Windhorse Publications; 2004.
15. Kabat-Zinn J. An outpatient program in behavioral medicine for chronic pain patients based on the practice of mindfulness meditation: theoretical considerations and preliminary results. Gen Hosp Psychiatry 1982;4(1):33–47.
16. Kabat-Zinn J, Lipworth L, Burney R. The clinical use of mindfulness meditation for the self-regulation of chronic pain. J Behav Med 1985;8(2):163–90.
17. Cherkin DC, Sherman KJ, Balderson BH, et al. Effect of mindfulness-based stress reduction vs cognitive behavioral therapy or usual care on back pain and functional limitations in adults with chronic low back pain: a randomized clinical trial. JAMA 2016; 315(12):1240–9.
18. Hilton L, Hempel S, Ewing BA, et al. Mindfulness meditation for chronic pain: systematic review and meta-analysis. Ann Behav Med 2017;51(2): 199–213.
19. Stanic JBJ, Danon N, Bondolfi G, et al. Adherence to standardized 8-week mindfulness-based interventions among women with breast or gynecological cancer: a scoping review. J Psychosocial Oncol Res Pract 2021;3(2):e048.
20. Ribeiro L, Atchley RM, Oken BS. Adherence to practice of mindfulness in novice meditators: practices chosen, amount of time practiced, and long-term effects following a mindfulness-based intervention. Mindfulness (N Y) 2018;9(2):401–11.
21. Agras WS. Understanding compliance with the medical regimen: the scope of the problem and a theoretical perspective. Arthritis Care Res 1989; 2(3):S2–7.
22. Kropotov JD. Chapter 2.2 - Alpha rhythms. In: Levy N, editor. Functional neuromarkers for psychiatry. San Diego (CA): Academic Press; 2016. p. 89–105.
23. Kropotov JD. Chapter 2.3 - Beta and gamma rhythms. In: Levy N, editor. Functional neuromarkers for psychiatry. San Diego (CA): Academic Press; 2016. p. 107–19.
24. Huber MT, Bartling J, Pachur D, et al. EEG responses to tonic heat pain. Exp Brain Res 2006; 173(1):14–24.
25. Wang MY, Bailey NW, Payne JE, et al. A systematic review of pain-related neural processes in expert and novice meditator. Mindfulness 2021;12(4): 799–814.
26. Jensen MP, Sherlin LH, Fregni F, et al. Baseline brain activity predicts response to neuromodulatory pain treatment. Pain Med 2014;15(12):2055–63.
27. Ratcliff CG, Prinsloo S, Chaoul A, et al. A randomized controlled trial of brief mindfulness meditation for women undergoing stereotactic breast biopsy. J Am Coll Radiol 2019;16(5):691–9.
28. Brown CA, Jones AKP. Meditation experience predicts less negative appraisal of pain: electrophysiological evidence for the involvement of anticipatory neural responses. Pain 2010;150(3):428–38.
29. Brown CA, Jones AK. Psychobiological correlates of improved mental health in patients with

musculoskeletal pain after a mindfulness-based pain management program. Clin J Pain 2013;29(3): 233–44.

30. Zeidan F, Grant JA, Brown CA, et al. Mindfulness meditation-related pain relief: evidence for unique brain mechanisms in the regulation of pain. Neurosci Lett 2012;520(2):165–73.

31. Zeidan F, Emerson NM, Farris SR, et al. Mindfulness meditation-based pain relief employs different neural mechanisms than placebo and sham mindfulness meditation-induced analgesia. J Neurosci 2015;35(46):15307–25.

32. Gard T, Hölzel BK, Sack AT, et al. Pain attenuation through mindfulness is associated with decreased cognitive control and increased sensory processing in the brain. Cereb Cortex 2012;22(11):2692–702.

33. Zeidan F, Martucci KT, Kraft RA, et al. Brain mechanisms supporting the modulation of pain by mindfulness meditation. J Neurosci 2011;31(14):5540–8.

34. Grant JA, Courtemanche J, Rainville P. A non-elaborative mental stance and decoupling of executive and pain-related cortices predicts low pain sensitivity in Zen meditators. Pain 2011;152(1):150–6.

35. Oshiro Y, Quevedo AS, McHaffie JG, et al. Brain mechanisms supporting discrimination of sensory features of pain: a new model. J Neurosci 2009; 29(47):14924–31.

36. Davis KD, Taylor SJ, Crawley AP, et al. Functional MRI of pain- and attention-related activations in the human cingulate cortex. J Neurophysiol 1997; 77(6):3370–80.

37. O'Doherty J, Kringelbach ML, Rolls ET, et al. Abstract reward and punishment representations in the human orbitofrontal cortex. Nat Neurosci 2001; 4(1):95–102.

38. Rolls ET, Grabenhorst F. The orbitofrontal cortex and beyond: from affect to decision-making. Prog Neurobiol 2008;86(3):216–44.

39. Jinich-Diamant A, Garland E, Baumgartner J, et al. Neurophysiological mechanisms supporting mindfulness meditation-based pain relief: an updated review. Curr Pain Headache Rep 2020; 24(10):56.

40. Morone NE, Greco CM, Moore CG, et al. A mind-body program for older adults with chronic low back pain: a randomized clinical trial. JAMA Intern Med 2016;176(3):329–37.

41. Zeidan F, Adler-Neal AL, Wells RE, et al. Mindfulness-meditation-based pain relief is not mediated by endogenous opioids. J Neurosci 2016;36(11): 3391–7.

42. Ruskin DA, Gagnon MM, Kohut SA, et al. A mindfulness program adapted for adolescents with chronic pain: feasibility, acceptability, and initial outcomes. Clin J Pain 2017;33(11):1019–29.

43. Taren AA, Gianaros PJ, Greco CM, et al. Mindfulness meditation training alters stress-related amygdala resting state functional connectivity: a randomized controlled trial. Soc Cogn Affect Neurosci 2015;10(12):1758–68.

44. Segal ZV, Dimidjian S, Beck A, et al. Outcomes of online mindfulness-based cognitive therapy for patients with residual depressive symptoms: a randomized clinical trial. JAMA Psychiatry 2020;77(6): 563–73.

45. Turner JA, Anderson ML, Balderson BH, et al. Mindfulness-based stress reduction and cognitive behavioral therapy for chronic low back pain: similar effects on mindfulness, catastrophizing, self-efficacy, and acceptance in a randomized controlled trial. Pain 2016;157(11):2434–44.

46. Case L, Adler-Neal AL, Wells RE, et al. The role of expectations and endogenous opioids in mindfulness-based relief of experimentally induced acute pain. Psychosom Med 2021;83(6):549–56.

47. Lindahl JR, Fisher NE, Cooper DJ, et al. The varieties of contemplative experience: a mixed-methods study of meditation-related challenges in Western Buddhists. PLoS One 2017;12(5): e0176239.

Financial Sustainability of Neuromodulation for Pain

Jason M. Schwalb, MD

KEYWORDS

- Neuromodulation • Pain • Financial sustainability • Cost effectiveness • Markov analysis • ICER
- QALY

KEY POINTS

- Neuromodulation, especially spinal cord stimulation, has significant evidence suggesting that it is more cost effective than continued medical management and traditional spine surgery.
- Many studies of cost effectiveness have limited applicability due to assumptions made in their development, differences in health care systems and shifting technologies and costs over time.
- There is a need for prospective registries in neuromodulation and alternative therapies that include analysis of cost effectiveness.

INTRODUCTION

When considering the financial sustainability of neuromodulation for pain, one needs to consider the varying costs involved with this therapy. These can include costs leading up to neuromodulation versus costs after neuromodulation is instituted; comparisons between different types of neuromodulation; comparisons between neuromodulation and conventional therapy; and comparisons between neuromodulation and other invasive modalities, such as spinal decompression with or without fusion. In addition, any consideration of cost also needs to take quality into account. Even if a therapy is expensive, it is considered cost-effective if it leads to significant increase in quality of life and economic productivity of the patient. This review considers these questions, methodologies used to assess them, and variations between different health delivery systems.

METHODOLOGY

Early studies tended to examine costs before an intervention and compare them with costs after an intervention. If the costs increase significantly, the intervention will not seem (on the surface) to be cost-effective. However, even if the costs of health care use decreased after the intervention, it is often unclear whether the costs would have gone down anyway because of the natural history of the disease decreasing in severity over time (regression to the mean). Patients are more likely to seek an intervention when their symptoms are at their worst.

The simplest way of looking at cost-effectiveness seems to be to examine costs of care within the structure of prospective, randomized controlled trials, but these may not reflect real life situations, because patients in clinical trials tend to receive more attention and care. They have avenues to reach research coordinators and clinicians, which can obviate expensive emergency department (ED) visits and imaging. Therefore, matched cohorts of patients where one group undergoes an intervention, and another similar group does not are often considered more representative of real life. This accounts for the natural history of the disease condition. However, there are often questions about whether the groups are adequately matched. There could be reasons that one group underwent the intervention, and the other did not that are not reflected in commonly used matched characteristics that are easily captured, such as age, pain severity, race, socioeconomic class, or International Classification of Diseases-10 code. It could even be that

Department of Neurosurgery, Henry Ford Medical Group, Detroit, MI, USA
E-mail address: jschwal1@hfhs.org

Neurosurg Clin N Am 33 (2022) 281–286
https://doi.org/10.1016/j.nec.2022.03.001
1042-3680/22/

the drive to seek the intervention or choose one intervention over another could positively influence outcome.

An additional issue is that costs vary among stakeholders.[1] Private insurers consider the cost of medical care, but governmental insurers may also consider loss of taxpayer revenue from inability to work and nonmedical costs, such as need for increased social support. Employers want their employees to return to work and not draw disability payments. Patients consider costs of insurance, copayments, and indirect costs, such as time that caregivers may need to take off work.

Even if the costs are higher for some period after the intervention, it may be perceived as being worthwhile for long-term improvement in quality of life. Quality of life is generally expressed as quality-adjusted life-years (QALYs), where a QALY of 1 is equivalent to 1 year of perfect health and a QALY of 0 is death.[2] There are standardized measures based on patient surveys, such as the EQ-5D (EuroQol, Rotterdam, The Netherlands), which are used to calculate QALYs.

QALYs are assigned to different outcomes. For example, the patient who gets 5 years of benefit from their spinal cord stimulator with significant improvement in pain and function is going to have a higher number of QALYs when compared with the patient who lost benefit at a year and then developed an infection, requiring explantation. Cost-effectiveness is generally expressed as the incremental cost-effectiveness ratio (ICER), defined as the difference in cost between two treatments divided by the difference in effects of the two treatments. Although the United States Affordable Care Act prohibited decisions on health insurance coverage based on cost per QALY, this is not true in other countries. Most modern industrialized nations are willing to pay $50,000 to $100,000 per QALY.

Decision trees and Markov models are developed to account for the probabilities of different outcomes of differing values. Incidences of different outcomes are varied as part of a sensitivity analysis to determine a threshold for willingness to pay (e.g., it might only make sense to cover the procedure if the complication rate can be brought lower than 5%).

Of course, the devil is in the details. There are different results for the same intervention for different indications. A therapy may not be cost-effective at 1 year but can be at 3 or 5 years (or vice versa), so duration of follow-up is paramount. Costs for treatment and implants can vary widely between countries: the average expense of a spinal cord stimulator system is CAN$21,595 in Canada and $32,882 in the United States with Medicare coverage.[3] Caution should be applied when referring to studies of cost-effectiveness that are more than 10 years old because of changes in pricing. In addition, other social issues can lead to differences in cost: the United States is an outlier in ED use. Imaging use and costs are higher in the United States. Conversely, higher rates of opioid use and abuse in the United States lead to increased disability and death, so an opioid-sparing modality, such as neuromodulation, may be particularly attractive.

SPINAL CORD STIMULATION

Most of the research done on cost-effectiveness for neuromodulation has focused on spinal cord stimulation (SCS), as nicely reviewed by Odonkor and colleagues.[3] Most analyses have been done for back and leg pain after spinal surgery, although there have also been some for complex regional pain syndrome (CRPS), peripheral arterial disease, refractory angina pectoris, neuropathic leg pain, and chronic back and leg pain without prior spinal surgery. In general, SCS was cost-effective when compared with conventional therapy, even with the higher implant and maintenance costs in the United States. There is reduction in postoperative use of physiotherapy, chiropractic treatment, massage therapy, injections, ED visits, imaging studies, and pharmacotherapy in the SCS group.[4] Despite the increased costs of rechargeable internal pulse generators (IPGs), they are generally cost-effective if the life expectancy of a primary cell is less than 4 years. The increased effectiveness and higher positive trial rate of some systems, such as those with 10-kHz stimulation relative to those with paresthesia-inducing stimulation paradigms, may make them cost-effective despite their increased cost.[5] However, these findings are somewhat suspect in that the data used to assess paresthesia-inducing stimulation were from 9 years before[6] with older technology.

Of note, there is evidence that delaying SCS therapy with nonoperative options tended to lead to decreased cost-effectiveness in addition to decreased efficacy. Patients with longer preimplant histories of pain had higher opioid use, and more frequent office visits and hospitalizations.

By examining insurance company data from 2000 to 2012 using the Truven Reuters MarketScan database (Truven Health Analytics, Ann Arbor, MI), Farber and colleagues[7] were able to identify 122,827 patients with failed back surgery syndrome with at least a year of continuous data. Truven data include inpatient and outpatient claims from 200 million patients with employer-

Total Cost Time Trend

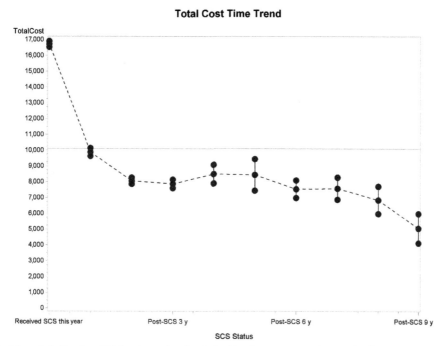

Fig. 1. Cost trends following SCS implantation for failed back surgery syndrome. (Farber SH, Han JL, Elsamadicy AA, et al. Long-term cost utility of spinal cord stimulation in patients with failed back surgery syndrome. *Pain Phys* 2017;20(6):E797-E805).[7]

based health insurance, Medicare, and Medicaid. About 4% of patients who had chronic pain after lumbar spinal surgery went on to have SCS systems implanted. Although the nature of the database precluded analysis of pain control and patient satisfaction, there was significant reduction in costs after SCS implantation, generally because of decreased health care use. The costs before implant were more than double in the subgroup who underwent SCS when compared with the conventional medical management (CMM) group, suggesting that they had more disabling pain that led to higher health care use. However, even at 1 year, the SCS group had much lower health care expenditures. These differences were maintained at 9 years after SCS implantation (**Fig. 1**).[8] It is unclear how many patients in the CMM group had expert care from pain physicians, while it is reasonable to assume that most, if not all, of those in the SCS patient group did. Therefore, it is difficult to parse whether the decreased costs associated with SCS were caused by more expert care from pain medicine physicians as opposed to the procedure itself.

Often the alternative to SCS is not CMM but repeat spinal surgery. In one systematic review,[9] 11 studies of cost-effectiveness in lumbar spinal surgery were found to be of adequate quality. At a population level, surgeries for decompression

were cost-effective relative to CMM at 1 year, but surgery for spondylolisthesis only became cost-effective at 4 years. However, as other studies have noted,[10] there is wide variability in costs and outcomes of lumbar spinal surgery.

The oft-cited trial by North and colleagues[11] from 2005 prospectively randomized patients with radicular symptoms after lumbar spinal surgery to either repeat spinal surgery or SCS. The patients did not have a progressive neurologic deficit and were not grossly unstable. SCS was superior in terms of opioid use and pain relief with lower neurologic morbidity and had a lower crossover rate to the other treatment modality. Economic analysis, at least within the UK National Health System, suggested that SCS confers an additional 0.98 QALYs when compared with repeat spinal surgery, for an ICER of £6392 per QALY. Spine surgeons tend to argue against the validity of these findings because of the small sample size in the trial (n = 50) at a single center and advances in the field since then, including better understanding of sagittal balance and improved surgical techniques. However, SCS has also advanced, and now features more complex lead design and different stimulation paradigms that have led to better results.[12,13] Although it may be difficult to organize and fund an updated prospective study of SCS versus repeat spine surgery, there is a need for registries that would enable cohort matching of such patients to update this prior analysis.

DORSAL ROOT GANGLION STIMULATION

In the industry-funded ACCURATE study, dorsal root ganglion (DRG) stimulation was compared with SCS with paresthesia-inducing stimulation paradigms in the treatment of CRPS types 1 and 2 of the lower extremities.[14] Subsequent analysis of the costs was based on MarketScan data,[15] with the assumption that the costs were the same for both technologies because they share a CPT code. The 10-year estimated costs of DRG stimulation ($153,992 ± $36,651) were higher than those associated with SCS ($128,269 ± $27,771) and CMM ($106,173 ± $27,005), mostly based on an estimate that the IPG for a DRG system would last 3.5 years and the rechargeable IPG for the SCS system would last 9 years. Clearly the costs of DRG and SCS are higher than CMM in this model, but the ICER was $34,695 per QALY gained with DRG over CMM, whereas the ICER of SCS compared with CMM was $22,084 per QALY. The difference in cost between DRG and SCS narrows because of the higher positive trial rate and increased efficacy of DRG stimulation versus SCS in the trial. When comparing DRG with SCS, the ICER was $68,095 per QALY. Thus, if cost is an issue and one considers willingness to pay as part of coverage decisions (ie, outside the United States), DRG is only favored over conventional SCS if one is willing to pay more than $68,000 per QALY. A cutoff of $50,000/QALY would favor SCS. Subsequent analyses with newer IPGs for DRG stimulation, with an estimated life of 6.5 years, make DRG much more cost-effective with an ICER of DRG versus SCS of $30,452/QALY.

However, the loss of efficacy rate and complication rate for DRG were based on the 12-month outcomes of the ACCURATE trial and expert opinion. Because this technology has not been available for 10 years, extrapolations were necessary. It was assumed that efficacy would remain stable from 12 months to 10 years. Despite clear evidence that many patients with CRPS improve over time with CMM,[16,17] costs in the CMM arm were assumed to be stable for 10 years. Thus, even though sensitivity analysis was carried out using a Monte Carlo simulation with 10,000 trials, many of the assumptions may make this analysis invalid. There is also no comparison of DRG versus paresthesia-free SCS stimulation paradigms. With advances in technology, much of the data may no longer be relevant.

PERIPHERAL NERVE STIMULATION

Peripheral nerve stimulation is an expanding field. Although first described by Scribonius Largus with Torpedo fish in 153 CE,[18] the modern era of implants for peripheral nerve stimulation began with Wall and Sweet[19] in 1967. Since then, most iterations involved directly exposing the nerve, wrapping a paddle electrode around the nerve,[18] and connecting the lead to an IPG. There were significant issues with scarring around nerves preventing normal sliding, and the potential need to cross joints to place an IPG. However, there are multiple new options for stimulation that do not involve IPGs and can be placed through a Touhy needle under fluoroscopic or ultrasound guidance.[20,21] The patient places a pad over a receiver to transmit energy to the system at much lower cost than an IPG. Because of the lack of an IPG, there is little financial justification for performing a trial before a permanent implant. Performing a lead placement with an externalized wire as a trial before implanting a permanent lead and receiver as permanent system essentially doubles the cost. In addition, because of concern about infection, the length of the trial and number of stimulation parameters that can be tried are limited.[22] Insurers are generally still requiring trials because of their lack of understanding of the finances. A cost-effectiveness analysis using claims data is sorely needed to rectify this situation.

Currently, the only available study on cost-effectiveness of peripheral nerve stimulation is for occipital nerve stimulation for cluster headache in a French registry.[23] Data for 3 months were extrapolated to 1 year with significant benefit versus CMM before implant. The average extrapolated total cost for 1 year was €1344 lower for the occipital nerve stimulation strategy with a gain of 0.28 QALY, resulting in an ICER of €4846/QALY. However, costs related to health care use could have gone down anyway because of regression to the mean. Characteristics of the French health care system may not be relevant to other countries.

DEEP BRAIN STIMULATION

The earliest examples of the use of deep brain stimulation in the 1950s were for pain.[24] However, the Food and Drug Administration withdrew approval for deep brain stimulation for pain in 1989. In response, Medtronic (Dublin, Ireland) sponsored two prospective trials to examine its efficacy. Although these trials were completed in 1993 and 1998, they were not reported until 2001, presumably because of the poor outcomes.[25] In general, only 20% of patients had positive results. The success rate could not be significantly improved by improving patient selection.[26] Thus, although the Affordable Care Act prohibits coverage decisions based on cost, one might surmise that the low success rate and high costs of this procedure has led to lack of coverage for these patients, despite the lack of more effective alternatives in a patient population for whom this is the last resort.

MOTOR CORTEX STIMULATION

Motor cortex stimulation (MCS) has been performed since 1988 for various types of unilateral face and arm deafferentation pain, with varying results. Despite being supported by two prospective randomized controlled trials,[27,28] the efficacy in reducing preoperative pain by greater than 40% is generally thought to be about 50%.[29] The costs of the initial procedure are high, because a craniotomy is generally involved and most clinicians perform an inpatient externalized trial before committing the patient to a permanent system with an IPG.

One way to increase the cost-effectiveness is to increase the likelihood of a successful trial. MCS is more effective for facial pain, phantom limb pain, and CRPS, compared with poststroke pain or pain associated with brachial plexus avulsion.[28] Machine learning has been used to identify preoperative characteristics to increase the likelihood of a positive response to 66%.[30] However, many would find it unpalatable to deny care based on gender, which is the most important factor in this dataset in predicting response, even more than response to repetitive transcranial magnetic stimulation.

Zaghi and colleagues[31] analyzed cost-effectiveness of MCS versus repetitive transcranial magnetic stimulation and transcranial direct current stimulation. Costs were estimated based on time, salary, rent, and hospitalization-related costs, but the sources are not clear. Claims data were not used. MCS was estimated at $42,000, which seems low. ICERs were expressed as cost per unit of Visual Analog Scale. Subsequent analysis has suggested that improvements in quality of life are not wholly dependent on reduction in numeric pain scores.[32] Given the methodologic problems of this article, not much can be said about the cost-effectiveness of MCS, even though this study favored MCS.

SUMMARY

Analyses of cost-effectiveness are important in driving coverage policies. Many types of neuromodulation have been found to be cost-effective when compared with continued, ineffective therapy or other interventions. However, care needs to be taken in looking at the assumptions used in model development. Although most studies look at 2-year outcomes, that may be insufficient for accurate analyses of cost-effectiveness. With advances in technology leading to better positive trial rates and efficacy, neuromodulation may become even more cost-effective over time. Registries that include patient-reported outcomes and financial data are needed to generate matched cohort trials that can more accurately compare outcomes and help direct resources effectively.

CLINICS CARE POINTS

- Be cautious of the assumptions used in cost analyses of medical or surgical interventions.
- View old data with out-of-date technology with skepticism when trying to compare to current practice.
- Consider how applicable a cost analysis is to your medical practice environment.

REFERENCES

1. Schwalb JM, Nerenz D. How do we measure quality in the treatment of pain? Congress Quarterly 2013; 14(2):13–4.
2. Sackett DL, Haynes RB, Guyatt GH, et al. Clinical epidemiology: a basic science for clinical medicine. 2nd edition. Boston (MA): Little, Brown, & Co; 1991.
3. Odonkor CA, Orman S, Orhurhu V, et al. Spinal cord stimulation vs conventional therapies for the treatment of chronic low back and leg pain: a systematic review of health care resource utilization and outcomes in the last decade. Pain Med 2019;20: 2479–94.
4. Kumar K, Rizvi S. Cost-effectiveness of spinal cord stimulation therapy in management of chronic pain. Pain Med 2013;14:1631–49.
5. Annemans L, Van Buyten JP, Smith T, et al. Cost effectiveness of a novel 10 kHz high-frequency spinal cord stimulation system in patients with failed back surgery syndrome (FBSS). J Long Term Eff Med Implants 2014;24:173–83.
6. Kumar K, Taylor RS, Jacques L, et al. The effects of spinal cord stimulation in neuropathic pain are sustained: a 24-month follow-up of the prospective randomized controlled multicenter trial of the effectiveness of spinal cord stimulation. Neurosurgery 2008;63:762–70.
7. Farber SH, Han JL, Elsamadicy AA, et al. Long-term cost utility of spinal cord stimulation in patients with failed back surgery syndrome. Pain Physician 2017; 20:E797–805.

8. Bell GK, Kidd D, North RB. Cost-effectiveness analysis of spinal cord stimulation in treatment of failed back surgery syndrome. J Pain Symptom Manage 1997;13:286–95.

9. Chang D, Zygourakis CC, Wadhwa H, et al. Systematic review of cost-effectiveness analyses in U.S. spine surgery. World Neurosurg 2020;142:e32–57.

10. Parker SL, Chotai S, Devin CJ, et al. Bending the cost curve-establishing value in spine surgery. Neurosurgery 2017;80:S61–9.

11. North RB, Kidd DH, Farrokhi F, et al. Spinal cord stimulation versus repeated lumbosacral spine surgery for chronic pain: a randomized, controlled trial. Neurosurgery 2005;56:98–106.

12. Kapural L. Letter: Comparison of 10-kHz high-frequency and traditional low-frequency spinal cord stimulation for the treatment of chronic back and leg pain: 24-month results from a multicenter randomized controlled pivotal trial. Neurosurgery 2017;80:E176–7.

13. Karri J, Orhurhu V, Wahezi S, et al. Comparison of spinal cord stimulation waveforms for treating chronic low back pain: systematic review and meta-analysis. Pain Physician 2020;23:451–60.

14. Deer TR, Levy RM, Kramer J, et al. Dorsal root ganglion stimulation yielded higher treatment success rate for complex regional pain syndrome and causalgia at 3 and 12 months: a randomized comparative trial. Pain 2017;158:669–81.

15. Mekhail N, Deer TR, Poree L, et al. Cost-effectiveness of dorsal root ganglion stimulation or spinal cord stimulation for complex regional pain syndrome. Neuromodulation 2021;24:708–18.

16. Kemler MA, de Vet HC, Barendse GA, et al. Effect of spinal cord stimulation for chronic complex regional pain syndrome type I: five-year final follow-up of patients in a randomized controlled trial. J Neurosurg 2008;108:292–8.

17. Kemler MA, de Vet HC, Barendse GA, et al. Spinal cord stimulation for chronic reflex sympathetic dystrophy: five-year follow-up. N Engl J Med 2006; 354:2394–6.

18. Slavin KV. History of peripheral nerve stimulation. Prog Neurol Surg 2011;24:1–15.

19. Wall PD, Sweet WH. Temporary abolition of pain in man. Science 1967;155:108–9.

20. Deer T, Pope J, Benyamin R, et al. Prospective, multicenter, randomized, double-blinded, partial crossover study to assess the safety and efficacy of the novel neuromodulation system in the treatment of patients with chronic pain of peripheral nerve origin. Neuromodulation 2016;19:91–100.

21. Deer TR, Naidu R, Strand N, et al. A review of the bioelectronic implications of stimulation of the peripheral nervous system for chronic pain conditions. Bioelectron Med 2020;6:9.

22. North RB, Calodney A, Bolash R, et al. Redefining spinal cord stimulation "trials": a randomized controlled trial using single-stage wireless permanent implantable devices. Neuromodulation 2020; 23:96–101.

23. Bulsei J, Leplus A, Donnet A, et al. Occipital nerve stimulation for refractory chronic cluster headache: a cost-effectiveness study. Neuromodulation 2021; 24:1083–92.

24. Schwalb JM, Hamani C. The history and future of deep brain stimulation. Neurotherapeutics 2008;5: 3–13.

25. Coffey RJ. Deep brain stimulation for chronic pain: results of two multicenter trials and a structured review. Pain Med 2001;2:183–92.

26. Hamani C, Schwalb JM, Rezai AR, et al. Deep brain stimulation for chronic neuropathic pain: long-term outcome and the incidence of insertional effect. Pain 2006;125:188–96.

27. Lefaucheur JP, Drouot X, Cunin P, et al. Motor cortex stimulation for the treatment of refractory peripheral neuropathic pain. Brain 2009;132:1463–71.

28. Hamani C, Fonoff ET, Parravano DC, et al. Motor cortex stimulation for chronic neuropathic pain: results of a double-blind randomized study. Brain 2021; 144:2994–3004.

29. Cruccu G, Garcia-Larrea L, Hansson P, et al. EAN guidelines on central neurostimulation therapy in chronic pain conditions. Eur J Neurol 2016;23: 1489–99.

30. Henssen D, Witkam RL, Dao J, et al. Systematic review and neural network analysis to define predictive variables in implantable motor cortex stimulation to treat chronic intractable pain. J Pain 2019;20:1015–26.

31. Zaghi S, Heine N, Fregni F. Brain stimulation for the treatment of pain: a review of costs, clinical effects, and mechanisms of treatment for three different central neuromodulatory approaches. J Pain Manag 2009;2:339–52.

32. Parravano DC, Ciampi DA, Fonoff ET, et al. Quality of life after motor cortex stimulation: clinical results and systematic review of the literature. Neurosurgery 2019;84:451–6.

Spinal Cord Stimulation
New Waveforms and Technology

Dennis London, MD*, Alon Mogilner, MD, PhD

KEYWORDS

- Spinal cord stimulation • Dorsal root ganglion stimulation • Chronic pain • Neuromodulation
- Emerging technologies • Closed-loop stimulation

KEY POINTS

- The authors review recent advances in the way spinal cord stimulation is delivered for chronic pain.
- They discuss high frequency, burst, and dorsal root ganglion stimulation.
- They preview emerging technologies, such as closed-loop and wireless stimulation.

INTRODUCTION

The decades-long use of spinal cord stimulation (SCS) for treating a variety of pain syndromes has now been validated by multiple randomized trials that confirm the benefit of SCS in well-selected patients as compared with traditional medical management.[1–6] However, these trials have found pain relief of approximately 50% in half of the patients. In addition, efficacy of pain relief can wane or be lost over time.[7–9] The fraction of patients who do not respond to therapy, the partial pain relief in those who do, and the loss of effect over time have led to the development of novel stimulation paradigms and technologies.

Traditional tonic SCS, the only form of SCS in routine clinical use through the first decade of the twenty-first century, uses continuous stimulation at 40 to 100 Hz using electrodes in the dorsal epidural space. Because of orthodromic stimulation of the dorsal columns, stimulation at these frequencies induces paresthesias in dermatomes that correspond to the location of stimulation, which is targeted to the location of the patients' pain. The pain relief itself is likely a combination of numerous mechanisms including but not limited to activation of inhibitory interneurons in the dorsal horn (i.e., the gate control theory).[5]

Innovations on this approach have been variations in the stimulation waveform or its location, the timing of its application, or the technology used to induce stimulation. In this article, the authors describe different waveforms that have been developed and their clinical results. They then discuss a variety of techniques for dorsal root ganglion stimulation before giving an overview of wireless and closed-loop technologies.

WAVEFORMS IN SPINAL CORD STIMULATION
Parameters of Stimulation

To explain the rapid expansion in stimulation waveforms, the authors first establish the basic terminology and physics of stimulation.[10,11] The tissue being stimulated acts as a capacitor in that it can store charge and as a resistor in that it can transmit charge. In SCS, an electric potential difference, also called a voltage, is applied between one or many pairs of electrodes; this results in an electric charge traveling through the tissue from the positive to the negative electrode. This traveling charge is called current.

When a voltage is initially applied, the tissue is uncharged and gradually accumulates a charge. This charge counteracts the voltage of the electrodes. If the voltage is kept constant, the current will decrease over time to an asymptotic nonzero value as shown in **Fig. 1**A. In contrast, current can be kept constant by increasing the voltage

Department of Neurosurgery, Center for Neuromodulation, NYU Langone Health, 550 First Ave, Suite 8S, New York, NY 10016, USA
* Corresponding author.
E-mail address: dennis.london@nyulangone.org

Neurosurg Clin N Am 33 (2022) 287–295
https://doi.org/10.1016/j.nec.2022.02.006

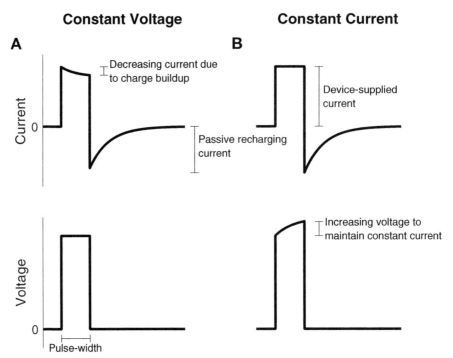

Fig. 1. Current and voltage waveform shapes for constant voltage (A) and constant current (B) modes of stimulation.

to counteract the accumulating charge on the tissue (**Fig. 1**B).

The voltage is applied between electrodes in pulses—that is for a defined length of time, the pulse width, which usually ranges from tens of microseconds up to 1 ms. The short length of pulses means that under constant current mode, the voltage does not change significantly, and under constant voltage mode, the voltage does not change significantly. Indeed, constant current and constant voltage modes of stimulation have been found to be clinically equivalent in traditional tonic SCS.[12] The amplitude of a pulse refers to the current under constant current mode and the voltage under constant voltage mode.

At the end of a pulse, the applied current and voltage are zero, and the built-up charge on the tissue redistributes to the device and to surrounding tissues. Charge thus travels in the opposite direction, generating negative current as measured by the generator, as shown in **Fig. 1**; this is analogous to the discharging of a capacitor and is often called passive recharge. Alternatively, the spinal cord stimulator may itself reverse the polarity of the electrodes to generate negative current; this is called active recharge.

In addition to the pulse width, amplitude, and shape, the final parameter that defines SCS is frequency—how many pulses are applied within a given length of time.

Tonic Spinal Cord Stimulation

Tonic SCS refers to the traditional form of SCS studied in most trials up until recently. As noted earlier, tonic stimulation uses continuous stimulation at 40 to 100 Hz with pulse widths on the order of hundreds of microseconds (**Fig. 2**A). These pulses are delivered under constant current or voltage settings and followed by passive recharge. Stimulation originates with an implantable pulse generator (IPG) that may or may not be rechargeable. This mode of stimulation induces paresthesias when applied with sufficient amplitude, which may vary based on the part of the spinal cord being stimulated as well as between individual patients based on their own unique neuroanatomy.

High-Frequency/High-Density Spinal Cord Stimulation

The frequency of nonresponse to tonic SCS therapy, particularly for back pain, and the decreasing effectiveness over time motivated the development of high-frequency SCS, initially deployed at 10 kHz with 30 μs pulses with active recharge,[13] as shown in **Fig. 2**D. The amplitude of stimulation is 1 to 5 mA, lower than tonic SCS and designed to be less than the threshold to cause paresthesias. The mechanisms of high-frequency stimulation are unclear (reviewed by Linderoth and Foreman[14]), but hypotheses include conduction

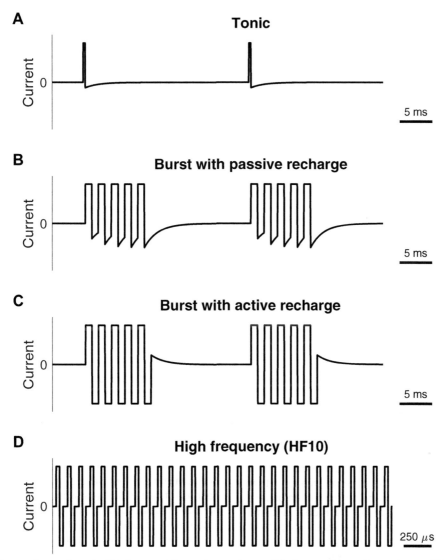

Fig. 2. Comparison of tonic (*A*), burst with passive recharge (*B*), burst with active recharge (*C*), and high-frequency (*D*) waveforms. Note the different timescale in (*D*).

blockade, inhibition of wide dynamic range neurons[15] and interneurons,[16] temperature increases,[17] and effects on glutamate uptake.[18]

This stimulation paradigm, known commercially as HF10 (Nevro, Redwood City, CA, USA), was demonstrated in a randomized clinical trial to afford pain relief in a greater proportion of patients than tonic SCS, especially for back pain,[19,20] with the response maintained for at least 3 years.[19,21,22] However, a different study found that the rate of response between tonic SCS and HF10 was not different.[23] High-frequency stimulation has also been shown to be effective for neck and arm pain.[24] HF10 stimulation is effective in more than half of patients who did not have a sufficient response to tonic SCS.[25,26]

The advent of HF10 has led to experimentation with high frequencies that are less than 10 kHz. The PROCO randomized controlled trial found equivalent pain control with 1, 4, 7, and 10 kHz stimulation,[27] whereas the randomized SCS Frequency Study found 5.88 kHz stimulation to be effective and 1.2 and 3.03 kHz stimulation to be no different from placebo.[28] The differing results are likely due to combination of factors including different devices (Boston Scientific in PROCO RCT and Nevro in SCS Frequency study), the use of a sham control in the SCS frequency study, different protocols and algorithms for stimulation program selection, and different inclusion criteria.

Some of these stimulation paradigms have been termed high-density or high-dose stimulation, referring to the current density or the "dose" of the electric charge. Current density can be increased in conventional spinal cord stimulators by increasing pulse width and frequency.[10] The frequency for high-density stimulation is commonly 1200 Hz, as this is the highest frequency that can be generated by conventional stimulators, but frequencies greater than 200 or 500 Hz can also be considered high density.[29–32] If amplitude is sufficiently decreased, these high current density settings are paresthesia-free. Paresthesia-free high-density stimulation settings can sometimes be used a salvage therapy when conventional tonic SCS becomes ineffective.[30,31,33–35]

Burst Spinal Cord Stimulation

The intrinsic bursting properties of thalamic neurons have inspired a different paresthesia-free waveform, known as burst stimulation.[36] In its most widespread form, known commercially as BurstDR (Abbott, Abbott Park, IL, USA), constant current stimulation is used at 500 Hz with 1 ms pulse width for periods of 10 ms, whose starts are spaced 25 ms apart (**Fig. 2**B). Thus, the frequency of the bursts, known as the interburst frequency, is 40 Hz. The stimulation is passively recharged; a small amount of passive recharge occurs during the 1 ms after each pulse during the burst. More complete passive recharge occurs in the 15 ms after each burst.

Several randomized placebo-controlled trials have shown burst stimulation is noninferior to tonic stimulation and may be better for certain aspects of pain. The first study by De Ridder and colleagues found similar responses in 15 patients for back and limb pain with tonic and burst stimulation, but burst stimulation was superior for "general pain" and affective pain scores,[37] consistent with increased modulation of dorsal anterior cingulate cortex by burst stimulation.[38] A second study of 15 patients found burst stimulation resulted in lower pain scores than tonic stimulation delivered at 500 Hz.[39] However, this is an atypical frequency for tonic stimulation, and burst stimulation seemed to have a similar effect compared with traditional ~40 Hz tonic stimulation although they were not directly compared. The larger SUNBURST trial found overall greater pain relief and a responder rate of 60% for burst compared with 51% for tonic stimulation[40]; however, these rates were not statistically compared, and the responder rate was defined as a 30% reduction in pain, lower than the usual 50% definition. Notably, all these trials included only patients who had a response to a trial of traditional tonic stimulation. However, several prospective studies have shown that burst stimulation seems to improve pain control for both responders and non-responders to tonic stimulation, suggesting it may be useful as rescue option.[41–43]

A variety of alternative burst stimulation paradigms have been deployed with variations in parameters, such as the frequency and the number of pulses in a burst.[44,45] These alternatives use active charge-balancing after each pulse (i.e., biphasic pulses, **Fig. 2**C). The importance of this point is controversial,[46,47] although biphasic and monophasic bursts may operate via different mechanisms.[48] However, prospective or randomized data for biphasic burst stimulation are lacking.

Intermittent Dosing and Combination Waveforms

Both high-frequency and burst stimulation result in pain control without paresthesias—patients do not know if stimulation is on at any given time; this led to the idea that stimulation may be halted entirely for certain times. Monophasic burst stimulation maintains its efficacy in a large fraction of patients even when it is only on for 30 seconds followed by 360 second off periods.[49,50] Many patients prefer this mode of stimulation, and the amount of off time preferred varies among patients. Similar results were recently demonstrated for HF10 stimulation with 20 second on periods and 120 second or 600 second off periods.[51]

Multiple devices are now also capable of cycling or overlaying different waveforms including combinations of paresthesia-causing waveforms and nonparesthesia causing waveforms.[35,52–55] One recent study found that the latter is preferred by a substantial fraction of patients.[35,54]

DORSAL ROOT GANGLION STIMULATION

Despite the aforementioned advances in SCS technologies, certain pathologies remain challenging to treat, including complex regional pain syndrome (CRPS)[56]; this has led to stimulation of the dorsal root ganglion stimulation (DRGS), which is achieved by percutaneous placement of leads in one or more intervertebral foramina.[57] DRGS is typically programmed at 10 to 50 Hz, with 30 to 1000 μs pulse width and amplitude around 1 mA. The significantly lower amplitude than for dorsal column SCS is likely due to the proximity of the lead to the site of action in DRGS.

The ongoing ACCURATE randomized trial has shown that DRGS provides pain relief in a greater proportion of patients with CRPS than tonic SCS.[56] This effect is durable at 1 year post-implant.

Interestingly, DRGS does not seem to depend on paresthesias although it does induce them. Despite its greater efficacy for CRPS, DRGS is associated with less paresthesia coverage of painful areas than SCS,[58] and more than one-third of patients become paresthesia-free over time without a decrease in pain control.[59]

Because DRGS is a newer modality, the diversity of waveforms available in SCS has not been replicated in DRGS although this is beginning. Recent work has shown that the frequency of DRGS can be tapered to 4 Hz without loss of pain relief,[60] and a small case series showed efficacy of 10 kHz DRGS using a wireless system.[61] In rats, monophasic burst stimulation of the DRG has similar efficacy to conventional DRGS in a model of painful diabetic peripheral neuropathy.[62] Findings are similar with tonic DRGS between 1 and 1000 Hz in rats.[63]

DORSAL NERVE ROOT STIMULATION

An alternative to SCS and DRGS for which there are limited clinical data is dorsal nerve root stimulation. In this technique, SCS leads are placed in the lateral dorsal epidural space over multiple nerve roots or partially within an intervertebral foramen and partially in the dorsal epidural space.[64] Several small trials have shown that this technique may have comparable efficacy to SCS.[65–67] Larger prospective and randomized trials are needed to further evaluate this technique.

CLOSED-LOOP STIMULATION

All technologies discussed thus far are open-loop—preprogrammed stimulation settings are executed by the system. However, pain varies with numerous factors including time of day, activity, and medication use. Furthermore, the response of pain to stimulation may vary as well. It is possible that stimulation may be optimized by allowing it to change its response to biologic systems; this is a closed-loop system.

One of the simplest variations in stimulation efficacy occurs with postural changes. The thickness of the cerebrospinal fluid layer between a spinal cord stimulator electrode and the dorsal columns decreases in the supine compared with the sitting or standing positions.[68] Thus, the stimulation threshold for paresthesias is higher when patients' are sitting or standing,[69] and patients often manually adjust their stimulation settings in different positions. The first closed-loop system used an accelerometer in the IPG to automatically sense position changes and adjust stimulation

accordingly, resulting in greater patient satisfaction in an unblinded randomized trial.[70]

Posture monitoring is an indirect way of measuring amplitude thresholds. Direct neural recordings would presumably be a more robust method. Indeed, evoked compound action potentials (ECAPs) can be recorded from SCS leads.[71] A novel closed-loop SCS system modulates the amplitude of stimulation in response to ECAPs recorded from the device.[72] In a blinded, randomized controlled trial, this form of closed-loop stimulation improved pain control in 82% of patients compared with 60% in open-loop stimulation, and this difference was maintained up to 1 year.[73] In a prospective, nonrandomized study, ECAP-based closed-loop stimulation maintained its efficacy for 2 years.[74]

The only parameter adjusted in a closed-loop fashion was the amplitude, but it is likely that future systems will adjust pulse width, frequency, and perhaps switch between any of the waveforms previously discussed in this article. Achieving this requires testing the ECAP response to these waveforms or developing novel biomarkers that can assess their efficacy.

WIRELESS STIMULATION

SCS systems have required connection of the lead to a pulse generator. The lead is externalized and connected to an external generator during the trial phase. A permanent system is placed including an implanted pulse generator if the trial is successful. Recently, a stimulation system has been developed in which stimulation settings and power are wirelessly transmitted using radiofrequency to a small, implanted receiver that wirelessly powers the electrode at frequencies up to 10 kHz[61]; this allows a pulse generator to be worn externally and recharged as needed and miniaturizes the implanted system. A trial that randomized participants to 10 kHz stimulation or low-frequency stimulation at traditional tonic, burst, or high-density settings found efficacy in both arms using wireless stimulation.[75] In several case reports, wireless stimulation has also been applied to DRGS[76] and peripheral nerve stimulation.[77]

SUMMARY

Technologies for SCS have massively diversified over the last decade. A plethora of new waveforms as well new techniques, such as DRGS have proved to be effective and allowed patients options if their initial therapy loses efficacy. High-frequency stimulation at 10 kHz and burst stimulation have become particularly widespread, and these are being further elaborated, although in which cases one is superior to the other has yet to be elucidated. Indeed, many devices now can provide multiple forms of stimulation so that this can be trialed in the individual patient. Trials are ongoing to determine the utility of mixing waveforms.

The parameter space of different waveforms is infinitely large, and searching for optimality is challenging. As our understanding of the pathophysiology of pain improves, targeting waveforms to specific pathways can narrow this search. Closed-loop stimulation is now available, and it may ultimately allow targeting stimulation paradigms toward specific biomarkers. The next phase of technology for SCS will involve discovering those biomarkers and harnessing devices to capture them.

CLINICS CARE POINTS

- Tonic SCS at 40 to 100 Hz is effective for many types of chronic pain but cannot effectively treat certain patients and often does not completely eliminate pain.

- High-frequency stimulation at 10 kHz provides patients with pain relief similar to traditional tonic SCS and may provide pain relief in patients who have failed traditional tonic stimulation.

- Burst stimulation seems to improve affective aspects of pain in patients for whom tonic stimulation is at least somewhat effective.

- High-frequency and burst stimulation have never been compared head-to-head, although they may both allow for salvage of patients in whom the other therapy has failed.

- Dorsal root ganglion stimulation is particularly effective for complex regional pain syndrome.

- Closed-loop stimulation is an emerging technology that is likely to allow more targeted stimulation, and potentially therapy tailored to specific pain pathways when they are active.

DISCLOSURE

D. London has nothing to disclose. A. Mogilner: Consultant: Medtronic, Abbott Medical, Boston Scientific. Grant Support: Medtronic, Abbott Medical

REFERENCES

1. De Vos CC, Meier K, Zaalberg PB, et al. Spinal cord stimulation in patients with painful diabetic neuropathy: A multicentre randomized clinical trial. Pain 2014;155(11):2426–31.

2. Kemler MA, Vet HCW de, Barendse GAM, et al. Effect of spinal cord stimulation for chronic complex regional pain syndrome Type I: five-year final follow-up of patients in a randomized controlled trial. J Neurosurg 2008;108(2):292–8.

3. Slangen R, Schaper NC, Faber CG, et al. Spinal Cord Stimulation and Pain Relief in Painful Diabetic Peripheral Neuropathy: A Prospective Two-Center Randomized Controlled Trial. Diabetes Care 2014; 37(11):3016–24.

4. Kumar K, Taylor RS, Jacques L, et al. The Effects of Spinal Cord Stimulation in Neuropathic Pain are Sustained: 24-Month Follow-Up of the Prospective Randomized Controlled Multicenter Trial of the Effectiveness of Spinal Cord Stimulation. Neurosurgery 2008;63(4):762–70.

5. Joosten EA, Franken G. Spinal cord stimulation in chronic neuropathic pain: mechanisms of action, new locations, new paradigms. Pain 2020;161:S104–13.

6. North RB, Kidd DH, Farrokhi F, et al. Spinal Cord Stimulation versus Repeated Lumbosacral Spine Surgery for Chronic Pain: A Randomized, Controlled Trial. Neurosurgery 2005;56(1):98–107.

7. Pope JE, Deer TR, Falowski S, et al. Multicenter Retrospective Study of Neurostimulation With Exit of Therapy by Explant. Neuromodulation Technol Neural Interf 2017;20(6):543–52.

8. Buyten J-P Van, Wille F, Smet I, et al. Therapy-Related Explants After Spinal Cord Stimulation: Results of an International Retrospective Chart Review Study. Neuromodulation Technol Neural Interf 2017; 20(7):642–9.

9. Hayek SM, Veizi E, Hanes M. Treatment-Limiting Complications of Percutaneous Spinal Cord Stimulator Implants: A Review of Eight Years of Experience From an Academic Center Database. Neuromodulation Technol Neural Interf 2015;18(7): 603–9.

10. Miller JP, Eldabe S, Buchser E, et al. Parameters of Spinal Cord Stimulation and Their Role in Electrical Charge Delivery: A Review. Neuromodulation Technol Neural Interf 2016;19(4):373–84.

11. Ortmanns M. Charge balancing in functional electrical stimulators: A comparative study. Proc - IEEE Int Symp Circuits Syst 2007;573–6.

12. Schade CM, Sasaki J, Schultz DM, et al. Assessment of Patient Preference for Constant Voltage and Constant Current Spinal Cord Stimulation. Neuromodulation Technol Neural Interf 2010;13(3): 210–7.

13. Russo M, Buyten J-P Van. 10-kHz High-Frequency SCS Therapy: A Clinical Summary. Pain Med Off J Am Acad Pain Med 2015;16(5):934.

14. Linderoth B, Foreman RD. Conventional and Novel Spinal Stimulation Algorithms: Hypothetical

Mechanisms of Action and Comments on Outcomes. Neuromodulation Technol Neural Interf 2017;20(6):525–33.

15. Cuellar JM, Alataris K, Walker A, et al. Effect of High-Frequency Alternating Current on Spinal Afferent Nociceptive Transmission. Neuromodulation Technol Neural Interf 2013;16(4):318–27.

16. Lee KY, Lee D, Kagan ZB, et al. Differential Modulation of Dorsal Horn Neurons by Various Spinal Cord Stimulation Strategies. Biomed 2021;9(5):568.

17. Zannou AL, Khadka N, Truong DQ, et al. Temperature increases by kilohertz frequency spinal cord stimulation. Brain Stimul 2019;12(1):62–72.

18. Liao WT, Tseng CC, Chia WT, et al. High-frequency spinal cord stimulation treatment attenuates the increase in spinal glutamate release and spinal miniature excitatory postsynaptic currents in rats with spared nerve injury-induced neuropathic pain. Brain Res Bull 2020;164:307–13.

19. Kapural L, Yu C, Doust MW, et al. Comparison of 10-kHz High-Frequency and Traditional Low-Frequency Spinal Cord Stimulation for the Treatment of Chronic Back and Leg Pain24-Month Results From a Multicenter, Randomized, Controlled Pivotal Trial. Neurosurgery 2016;79(5):667–77.

20. Kapural L, Yu C, Doust MW, et al. Novel 10-kHz High-frequency Therapy (HF10 Therapy) Is Superior to Traditional Low-frequency Spinal Cord Stimulation for the Treatment of Chronic Back and Leg PainThe SENZA-RCT Randomized Controlled Trial. Anesthesiology 2015;123(4):851–60.

21. Al-Kaisy A, Van Buyten J-P, Smet I, et al. Sustained Effectiveness of 10 kHz High-Frequency Spinal Cord Stimulation for Patients with Chronic, Low Back Pain: 24-Month Results of a Prospective Multicenter Study. Pain Med 2014;15(3):347–54.

22. Al-Kaisy A, Palmisani S, Smith TE, et al. Long-Term Improvements in Chronic Axial Low Back Pain Patients Without Previous Spinal Surgery: A Cohort Analysis of 10-kHz High-Frequency Spinal Cord Stimulation over 36 Months. Pain Med 2018;19(6):1219–26.

23. De Andres J, Monsalve-Dolz V, Fabregat-Cid G, et al. Prospective, Randomized Blind Effect-on-Outcome Study of Conventional vs High-Frequency Spinal Cord Stimulation in Patients with Pain and Disability Due to Failed Back Surgery Syndrome. Pain Med 2017;18(12):2401–21.

24. Amirdelfan K, Vallejo R, Benyamin R, et al. High-Frequency Spinal Cord Stimulation at 10 kHz for the Treatment of Combined Neck and Arm Pain: Results From a Prospective Multicenter Study. Neurosurgery 2020;87(2):176–85.

25. Kapural L, Sayed D, Kim B, et al. Retrospective Assessment of Salvage to 10 kHz Spinal Cord Stimulation (SCS) in Patients Who Failed Traditional SCS

Therapy: RESCUE Study. J Pain Res 2020;13:2861–7.

26. Tous NC, Corral CS, García IMO, et al. High-frequency spinal cord stimulation as rescue therapy for chronic pain patients with failure of conventional spinal cord stimulation. Eur J Pain 2021;25(7):1603–11.

27. Thomson SJ, Tavakkolizadeh M, Love-Jones S, et al. Effects of Rate on Analgesia in Kilohertz Frequency Spinal Cord Stimulation: Results of the PROCO Randomized Controlled Trial. Neuromodulation Technol Neural Interf 2018;21(1):67–76.

28. Al-Kaisy A, Palmisani S, Pang D, et al. Prospective, Randomized, Sham-Control, Double Blind, Crossover Trial of Subthreshold Spinal Cord Stimulation at Various Kilohertz Frequencies in Subjects Suffering From Failed Back Surgery Syndrome (SCS Frequency Study). Neuromodulation Technol Neural Interf 2018;21(5):457–65.

29. Goudman L, De Smedt A, Eldabe S, et al. High-dose spinal cord stimulation for patients with failed back surgery syndrome: a multicenter effectiveness and prediction study. Pain 2021;162(2):582–90.

30. Provenzano DA, Rebman J, Kuhel C, et al. The Efficacy of High-Density Spinal Cord Stimulation Among Trial, Implant, and Conversion Patients: A Retrospective Case Series. Neuromodulation Technol Neural Interf 2017;20(7):654–60.

31. Sweet J, Badjatiya A, Tan D, et al. Paresthesia-Free High-Density Spinal Cord Stimulation for Postlaminectomy Syndrome in a Prescreened Population: A Prospective Case Series. Neuromodulation Technol Neural Interf 2016;19(3):260–7.

32. Peeters JB, Raftopoulos C. Tonic, Burst, High-Density, and 10-kHz High-Frequency Spinal Cord Stimulation: Efficiency and Patients' Preferences in a Failed Back Surgery Syndrome Predominant Population. Review of Literature. World Neurosurg 2020;144:e331–40.

33. Wille F, Breel JS, Bakker EWP, et al. Altering Conventional to High Density Spinal Cord Stimulation: An Energy Dose-Response Relationship in Neuropathic Pain Therapy. Neuromodulation Technol Neural Interf 2017;20(1):71–80.

34. North J, Loudermilk E, Lee A, et al. Outcomes of a Multicenter, Prospective, Crossover, Randomized Controlled Trial Evaluating Subperception Spinal Cord Stimulation at ≤1.2 kHz in Previously Implanted Subjects. Neuromodulation Technol Neural Interf 2020;23(1):102–8.

35. Andrade P, Heiden P, Visser-Vandewalle V, et al. 1.2 kHz High-Frequency Stimulation as a Rescue Therapy in Patients With Chronic Pain Refractory to Conventional Spinal Cord Stimulation. Neuromodulation Technol Neural Interf 2021;24(3):540–5.

36. De Ridder D, Vanneste S, Plazier M, et al. Burst Spinal Cord StimulationToward Paresthesia-Free Pain Suppression. Neurosurgery 2010;66(5):986–90.

37. Dirk DR, Mark P, Niels K, et al. Burst spinal cord stimulation for limb and back pain. World Neurosurg 2013;80(5). https://doi.org/10.1016/J.WNEU.2013.01.040.

38. Yearwood T, Ridder D De, Yoo H Bin, et al. Comparison of Neural Activity in Chronic Pain Patients During Tonic and Burst Spinal Cord Stimulation Using Fluorodeoxyglucose Positron Emission Tomography. Neuromodulation Technol Neural Interf 2020;23(1):56–63.

39. Schu S, Slotty PJ, Bara G, et al. A Prospective, Randomised, Double-blind, Placebo-controlled Study to Examine the Effectiveness of Burst Spinal Cord Stimulation Patterns for the Treatment of Failed Back Surgery Syndrome. Neuromodulation Technol Neural Interf 2014;17(5):443–50. https://doi.org/10.1111/NER.12197.

40. Deer T, Slavin KV, Amirdelfan K, et al. Success Using Neuromodulation With BURST (SUNBURST) Study: Results From a Prospective, Randomized Controlled Trial Using a Novel Burst Waveform. Neuromodulation Technol Neural Interf 2018;21(1):56–66.

41. Vos CC de, Bom MJ, Vanneste S, et al. Burst Spinal Cord Stimulation Evaluated in Patients With Failed Back Surgery Syndrome and Painful Diabetic Neuropathy. Neuromodulation Technol Neural Interf 2014;17(2):152–9.

42. De Ridder D, Lenders MWPM, De Vos CC, et al. A 2-center comparative study on tonic versus burst spinal cord stimulation: Amount of responders and amount of pain suppression. Clin J Pain 2015;31(5):433–7.

43. Courtney P, Espinet A, Mitchell B, et al. Improved Pain Relief With Burst Spinal Cord Stimulation for Two Weeks in Patients Using Tonic Stimulation: Results From a Small Clinical Study. Neuromodulation Technol Neural Interf 2015;18(5):361–6.

44. Ahmed S, Yearwood T, Ridder D De, et al. Burst and high frequency stimulation: underlying mechanism of action. Expert Rev Med Devices 2017;15(1):61–70.

45. Clingan JA, Patel A, Maher DP. Survey of Spinal Cord Stimulation Hardware Currently Available for the Treatment of Chronic Pain in the United States. Front Pain Res 2020;0:4. https://doi.org/10.3389/FPAIN.2020.572907.

46. Ridder D De, Vancamp T, Falowski SM, et al. All bursts are equal, but some are more equal (to burst firing): burstDR stimulation versus Boston burst stimulation. Expert Rev Med Devices 2020;17(4):289–95.

47. Meuwissen KPV, Gu JW, Zhang TC, et al. Response to: Fundamental Differences in Burst Stimulation Waveform Design: Eliminating Confusion in the Marketplace. Neuromodulation Technol Neural Interf 2018;21(7):721–2.

48. Chakravarthy K, Fishman MA, Zuidema X, et al. Mechanism of Action in Burst Spinal Cord Stimulation: Review and Recent Advances. Pain Med 2019;20(Supplement_1):S13–22.

49. Deer TR, Patterson DG, Baksh J, et al. Novel Intermittent Dosing Burst Paradigm in Spinal Cord Stimulation. Neuromodulation Technol Neural Interf 2021;24(3):566–73.

50. Vesper J, Slotty P, Schu S, et al. Burst SCS Microdosing Is as Efficacious as Standard Burst SCS in Treating Chronic Back and Leg Pain: Results From a Randomized Controlled Trial. Neuromodulation Technol Neural Interf 2019;22(2):190–3.

51. Provenzano D, Tate J, Gupta M, et al. Pulse Dosing of 10 kHz Paresthesia-Independent Spinal Cord Stimulation Provides Same Efficacy with Substantial Reduction of Device Recharge Time. Pain Med 2021. https://doi.org/10.1093/PM/PNAB288.

52. Haider N, Ligham D, Quave B, et al. Spinal Cord Stimulation (SCS) Trial Outcomes After Conversion to a Multiple Waveform SCS System. Neuromodulation Technol Neural Interf 2018;21(5):504–7.

53. Duse G, Reverberi C, Dario A. Effects of Multiple Waveforms on Patient Preferences and Clinical Outcomes in Patients Treated With Spinal Cord Stimulation for Leg and/or Back Pain. Neuromodulation Technol Neural Interf 2019;22(2):200–7.

54. Kalleward JW, Jose Franscio P-S, Pasquale DN, et al. Real-World Outcomes Using a Spinal Cord Stimulation Device Capable of Combination Therapy for Chronic Pain: A European, Multicenter Experience. J Clin Med 2021;10(18). https://doi.org/10.3390/JCM10184085.

55. Hagedorn JM, Layno-Moses A, Sanders DT, et al. Overview of HF10 spinal cord stimulation for the treatment of chronic pain and an introduction to the Senza Omnia™ system. Pain Manag 2020;10(6):367–76.

56. Deer TR, Levy RM, Kramer J, et al. Dorsal root ganglion stimulation yielded higher treatment success rate for complex regional pain syndrome and causalgia at 3 and 12 months: A randomized comparative trial. Pain 2017;158(4):669–81.

57. Liem L, Russo M, Huygen FJPM, et al. A Multicenter, Prospective Trial to Assess the Safety and Performance of the Spinal Modulation Dorsal Root Ganglion Neurostimulator System in the Treatment of Chronic Pain. Neuromodulation Technol Neural Interf 2013;16(5):471–82.

58. Deer TR, Levy RM, Kramer J, et al. Comparison of Paresthesia Coverage of Patient's Pain: Dorsal Root Ganglion vs. Spinal Cord Stimulation. An ACCURATE Study Sub-Analysis. Neuromodulation Technol Neural Interf 2019;22(8):930–6.

59. Mekhail N, Deer TR, Kramer J, et al. Paresthesia-Free Dorsal Root Ganglion Stimulation: An ACCURATE Study Sub-Analysis. Neuromodulation Technol Neural Interf 2020;23(2):185–95.

60. Chapman KB, Yousef TA, Vissers KC, et al. Very Low Frequencies Maintain Pain Relief From Dorsal Root

Ganglion Stimulation: An Evaluation of Dorsal Root Ganglion Neurostimulation Frequency Tapering. Neuromodulation Technol Neural Interf 2021;24(4): 746–52.

61. Billet B, Hanssens K, Coster O De, et al. Wireless high-frequency dorsal root ganglion stimulation for chronic low back pain: A pilot study. Acta Anaesthesiol Scand 2018;62(8):1133–8.

62. Franken G, Debets J, Joosten EAJ. Dorsal Root Ganglion Stimulation in Experimental Painful Diabetic Peripheral Neuropathy: Burst vs. Conventional Stimulation Paradigm. Neuromodulation Technol Neural Interf 2019;22(8):943–50.

63. Koetsier E, Franken G, Debets J, et al. Dorsal Root Ganglion Stimulation in Experimental Painful Diabetic Polyneuropathy: Delayed Wash-Out of Pain Relief After Low-Frequency (1Hz) Stimulation. Neuromodulation Technol Neural Interf 2020;23(2): 177–84.

64. Haque R, Winfree CJ. Spinal nerve root stimulation. Neurosurg Focus 2006;21(6):1–7.

65. Levine AB, Parrent AG, MacDougall KW. Stimulation of the spinal cord and dorsal nerve roots for chronic groin, pelvic, and abdominal pain. Pain Physician 2016;19(6):405–12.

66. Levine AB, Parrent AG, Macdougall KW. Cervical spinal cord and dorsal nerve root stimulation for neuropathic upper limb pain. Can J Neurol Sci 2017;44(1):83–9.

67. Abbass M, Santyr BG, Parrent AG, et al. Paresthesia-Free Spinal Nerve Root Stimulation for the Treatment of Chronic Neuropathic Pain. Neuromodulation Technol Neural Interf 2020;23(6):831–7.

68. Barolat G. Epidural Spinal Cord Stimulation: Anatomical and Electrical Properties of the Intraspinal Structures Relevant to Spinal Cord Stimulation and Clinical Correlations. Neuromodulation Technol Neural Interf 1998;1(2):63–71.

69. Olin JC, Kidd DH, North RB. Postural Changes in Spinal Cord Stimulation Perceptual Thresholds. Neuromodulation Technol Neural Interf 1998;1(4): 171–5.

70. David S, Lynn W, Peter K, Urfan D, et al. Sensor-driven position-adaptive spinal cord stimulation for chronic pain. Pain Physician 2012;15(1):1–12.

71. Parker JL, Karantonis DM, Single PS, et al. Compound action potentials recorded in the human spinal cord during neurostimulation for pain relief. Pain 2012;153(3):593–601.

72. Russo M, Cousins MJ, Brooker C, et al. Effective Relief of Pain and Associated Symptoms With Closed-Loop Spinal Cord Stimulation System: Preliminary Results of the Avalon Study. Neuromodulation Technol Neural Interf 2018;21(1):38–47.

73. Mekhail N, Levy RM, Deer TR, et al. Long-term safety and efficacy of closed-loop spinal cord stimulation to treat chronic back and leg pain (Evoke): a double-blind, randomised, controlled trial. Lancet Neurol 2020;19(2):123–34.

74. Brooker C, Russo M, Cousins MJ, et al. ECAP-Controlled Closed-Loop Spinal Cord Stimulation Efficacy and Opioid Reduction Over 24-Months: Final Results of the Prospective, Multicenter, Open-Label Avalon Study. Pain Pract 2021;21(6):680–91.

75. Bolash R, Creamer M, Rauck R, et al. Wireless High-Frequency Spinal Cord Stimulation (10 kHz) Compared with Multiwaveform Low-Frequency Spinal Cord Stimulation in the Management of Chronic Pain in Failed Back Surgery Syndrome Subjects: Preliminary Results of a Multicenter, Prospective Randomized Controlled Study. Pain Med 2019; 20(10):1971–9.

76. Billet B, Wynendaele R, Vanquathem NE. Wireless neuromodulation for chronic back pain: Delivery of high-frequency dorsal root ganglion stimulation by a minimally invasive technique. Case Rep Med 2017;2017. https://doi.org/10.1155/2017/4203271.

77. Herschkowitz D, Kubias J. A case report of wireless peripheral nerve stimulation for complex regional pain syndrome type-I of the upper extremity: 1 year follow up. Scand J Pain 2019;19(4):829–35.

Closed-Loop Systems in Neuromodulation
Electrophysiology and Wearables

Thiago S. Montenegro, MD[a,b],*, Rushna Ali, MD[a,b],
Jeffrey E. Arle, MD, PhD[c,d,e]

KEYWORDS

• Closed-loop systems • Neuromodulation • Spinal cord stimulator • Wearable

KEY POINTS

• Most currently available neuromodulation techniques for pain work through an open-loop system delivering a fixed amplitude, pulse train, frequency, and pulse width, providing a preprogrammed fixed output, according to a programmed setting.
• The distance between the epidural space, where electrodes are placed with SCS, and the target of the stimulation in a dynamic body, can change because of physiologic conditions like posture, heart rate, and breathing.
• The closed-loop system in spinal cord neuromodulation consists of an integrated system that records real-time electrophysiological activity in the form of evoked compound action potentials (ECAPs) and uses it in a feedback mechanism to adjust stimulus output.
• Wearables represent newly developed technologies that have gained traction in recent years and were further popularized during the COVID-19 pandemic in different areas of medicine. Their application in pain management is still developing but promising.

INTRODUCTION

Pain is traditionally classified as nociceptive, neuropathic, and psychogenic. Nociceptive pain is essentially the unpleasant perception of a localized stimulation through nociceptors, while neuropathic pain is a result of a dysfunction of the signal transmission through nociceptive neurons, and psychogenic pain is the result of a psychiatric disorder not related to damage or stimuli to the affected site. Pain is a perceptual experience associated with unpleasant sensory and emotional experience, and the comprehension of the anatomy and physiology of its process is essential to better understanding of mechanisms of action of spinal cord stimulators, and more specifically closed-loop neuromodulation of pain.[1-3] The pain pathway begins with a transduction process, involving activation of peripheral nociceptors that are specific for the nature of each type of painful stimulus (chemical, mechanical, and thermal).[3,4] The transmission process of pain from free nerve endings to second-order neurons within the dorsal horn of the spinal cord occurs through 2 different pathways, a fast-sharp pain pathway and a slow-chronic pain pathway.[4-6]

Two different fibers are responsible for transmitting different types of pain. Small-type Aδ fibers are myelinated, mechanothermal fibers

No portion of the paper has been presented previously, published, or submitted for review in any other journal.
[a] Department of Neurosciences, Spectrum Health Medical Group, Grand Rapids, MI, USA; [b] Michigan State University, Grand Rapids, MI, USA; [c] Department of Neurosurgery, Beth Israel Deaconess Medical Center, Boston, MA, USA; [d] Department of Neurosurgery, Harvard Medical School, Boston, MA, USA; [e] Department of Neurosurgery, Mount Auburn Hospital, Cambridge, MA, USA
* Corresponding author. Department of Neurosciences, Spectrum Health Medical Group, 100 Michigan Street Northeast, Grand Rapids, MI 49503.
E-mail address: thiago.scharthmontenegro@spectrumhealth.org

responsible for carrying fast-sharp pain signals with a conduction speed that varies from 2 to 30 m/s. Type C fibers, the second type, are not myelinated and are responsible for the slow-chronic pain pathway, with conduction speed that varies from 0.5 to 2 m/s, mostly stimulated by chemical stimulation. Aδ fibers terminate within the lamina marginalis of the dorsal horn, secrete glutamate, and excite the second-order neurons of the spinothalamic tract that carry nociceptive information to the reticular areas of the brain stem and to the ventrobasal complex and ventral posterior nuclear group of the thalamus. The type C fibers terminate within the substantia gelatinosa, more specifically laminae II and III; secrete glutamate and substance P; and communicate through short fiber neurons to lamina V that projects to the reticular nuclei of the brain stem, tectal area of the mesencephalon, periaqueductal gray region, and the intralaminar and ventrolateral nuclei of the thalamus. Third-order neurons project to the somatosensory cortex, mediating perception of the intensity, localization, duration, and emotional components of pain.[4,5]

Three different innate endogenous mechanisms of pain modulation and 3 anatomic structures are important to this neural processing. Innate mechanisms include the segmental inhibition of pain forming the basis of the gate control theory of pain, the descending inhibitory system, and the endogenous opiate system.

Spinal cord stimulators (SCS) have been used as a therapeutic option to treat refractory chronic axial and limb pain for nearly 50 years after the seminal work by Melzack and Wall.[7] The most important concept to understand mechanism of action of SCS is the segmental inhibition of pain. It is known that the activation of the large, myelinated Aβ fibers responsible to transport nonnoxious sense touch stimuli cause inhibition of pain activity from slower unmyelinated C fibers through activation of inhibitory interneurons at the laminae III and IV causing local lateral inhibition in the spinal cord, modulating transmission of pain information. The Aβ are preferentially activated over smaller unmyelinated fibers given their lower thresholds for firing action potentials, and activating these fibers is one of the mechanisms SCSs use to modulate pain through the creation of an electric field that triggers retrograde action potentials, preferentially activating these large Aβ dorsal column axons[3,4,7,8] The concept that spinal cord structures are responsible for a gate control system that modulates the afferent patterns of pain before transmission to the brain led to a range of possible interventions and options to treat pain by neuromodulating the transmitting information.

These first devices, dorsal column stimulators, achieve pain relief with induced paresthesia as a secondary side effect of stimulating these touch- and vibration-carrying fibers.[8–12]

Another mechanism of pain modulation consists of the descending inhibitory system that originates on the cortical and subcortical areas. The noradrenergic pathway originates at the locus coeruleus and stimulates adrenergic receptors at the dorsal horn of the spinal cord, reducing the secretion of substance P and increasing the concentration of gamma-aminobutyric acid (GABA), thereby inhibiting pain-afferent pathways. The serotoninergic descending pathway originates at the nucleus raphe magnus and can be either inhibitory, activating 5-HT1A and 5-HT7 receptors, or excitatory, activating 5-HT2A and 5-HT3 receptors.[3,13,14] A third mechanism of pain modulation consists of the endogenous opioid system, where the breakdown products from large proteins (pro-opiomelanocortin, proenkephalin, and prodynorphin) produce opioid-like substances (β -endorphin, dynorphin, leu-enkephalin, met-enkephalin, among others) that are found in different regions of the nervous system, inhibiting pain pathways.[3–5]

The distance between the epidural SCS electrodes and the target neural fibers of the spinal cord is variable and depends on dorsal CSF column distance and spinal cord movement within the spinal canal, which can occur with even minimal physiologic movements like the cardiorespiratory cycle and changes in abdominal and thoracic pressures with coughing and postural changes. Additionally, it can generate asymmetrical recruitment by the SCS ,considering that the density of the current with SCS varies with the inverse of the distance between the electrode and spinal cord squared.[15–17] The width of the dorsal column of CSF has been demonstrated to have a wide variability with postural changes, with its thickness increasing by up to 2 times between the supine and prone positions.[15,18,19] These variations can cause understimulation or overstimulation of the target neural fibers if the SCS current is set in a fixed output.

All current SCS systems work through an open-loop system delivering a fixed amplitude, pulse train, frequency, and pulse width, providing a pre-programmed fixed output to the spinal cord, according to a programmed setting. However, the challenge of a steady control of pain in a dynamic body exists because of the changing distance between the stimulating electrodes and their spinal cord target, and consequently, the current reaching the spinal cord varies moment to moment.[16,20] In order to minimize this positional effect, Schultz and colleagues proposed a sensor-driven, position-adaptive stimulator that, with the aid of an accelerometer located in the pulse generator, delivers preprogrammed fixed output stimulation based on a sliding scale varying with gross postural changes.[16,20] This has proven to be a valuable advance in neuromodulation to address the common complaint from patients who felt discomfort with certain position changes and led them to manually adjust settings in situations without benefit. Yet the stimulation output varies based on postural change and not on how much current is reaching the spinal cord, still resulting in substantial variation in spinal cord activation.[20] Closed-loop systems were developed in this context.

A closed-loop system in spinal cord neuromodulation consists of components that record real-time electrophysiological activity in the form of evoked compound action potentials (ECAPs) and uses this information in a feedback mechanism to make a newly calculated stimulus output after each pulse, keeping the ECAP amplitude close to the target amplitude.[16,20,21] Recent studies have demonstrated that closed-loop stimulation results in fewer adverse effects, and increased efficacy and clinical benefit of neurostimulation.[16,22,23]

The Avalon Study, the Evoke Trial, and Clinical Evidence of Closed-Loop Efficacy

ECAPs are "the sum of multiple action potentials that result from activation of multiple nerve fibers by an electrical stimulus."[20] When measured at the dorsal column of the spinal cord, ECAPs are essentially a measure that represents the degree of the dorsal column stimulation and provides essential information to close the loop of neuromodulation through SCS. After a specific stimulus is delivered to the target through the SCS, ECAPs provide the response of the dorsal column to the stimulation giving the measure of activity.[24,25] The real-time availability of the number of fibers being recruited translated into the ECAPs provides the closed-loop systems the ability to automatically self-regulate the nature of the stimulus to meet the optimal stimulation settings within the therapeutic window set by the programmer.

The information in real time of the degree of the dorsal column stimulation enables an immediate correction of the stimulus delivered to the target, minimizing the difference between measured ECAP and target ECAPs, maximizing the amount of time under consistent spinal cord stimulation, and studies have demonstrated better pain control through this approach.[21,24]

Since the first experiments to measure ECAP in order to use it to guide SCS feedback control,

some animal clinical models have been evaluated and demonstrated superiority in pain control in comparison with open-loop fixed-input systems.[25-27] In 2015, the Avalon study started to enroll individuals for the first prospective, multicenter, single-arm study to evaluate the safety and efficacy of a closed-loop SCS system in humans, and its results from the 6-month, 12-month, and 24-month follow-ups have demonstrated significant improvements in pain control. After 24 months of the SCS implantation, 89.5% of patients reported achieving at least 50% pain reduction, while 68.5% of patients reported achieving at least 80% pain reduction.[21,28,29]

The Evoke trial is the first prospective multicenter, double-blind, randomized controlled trial comparing the efficacy and measuring spinal cord activation of open-loop fixed-output SCS and ECAP-controlled closed-loop SCS in patients with chronic, intractable back and leg pain. After 12 months of follow-up, patients who were in the closed-loop arm of the study were found to have greater spinal cord activation and greater pain relief, and significant benefit for quality of life improvement when compared with the open-loop group. The trial did demonstrate that 83.1% of the patients in the closed-loop arm of the study had 50% or greater reduction in overall back and leg pain with no increase in pain medications, compared with 61.0% in the open-loop group. In addition, patients in the closed-loop arm of the study spent 95.2% of the time within the therapeutic window, while patients in the open-loop group just spent 47.9% of the time within the stipulated therapeutic window.[20] Although promising, the Evoke trial was not free from criticism, and concerns were raised about possible measurement bias, the accuracy of the report, lack of a placebo group, long-term efficacy, and safety, given the short duration of follow-up.[30,31]

Transcutaneous Electrical Nerve Stimulation and Percutaneous Tibial Nerve Stimulation

Closed-loop stimulation has been implemented in settings other than SCS. Closed-loop neuromodulation applied to peripheral nerve instead of the spinal cord uses low-voltage transcutaneous electrical nerve stimulation (TENS) in different settings such as tremor modulation in Parkinson disease[32] and treatment of overactive bladder syndrome (OBS).[33] Percutaneous tibial nerve stimulation (PTNS) has been used to manage OBS since 1999, delivering fixed parameter settings. In the past years, the Bluewind RENOVA system, which is a wireless battery-free tibial nerve stimulation system, brought the closed-loop technology to the treatment of overactive bladder. The system ensures that the energy transferred from the external control unit (ECU) to the implant is stable throughout the treatment sessions within the pulse width and amplitude range set up by the clinician programmer.[33]

RATIONALE FOR THE USE OF CLOSED-LOOP NEUROMODULATION

Closed-loop systems may provide some advantages compared with open-loop fixed-output neuromodulation systems. The time-sensitive responsiveness and the capacity to adapt the neuromodulation response to unpredictable parameters are advantages of closed-loop SCS. In order to deliver an intervention in a timely manner, providing better state-dependent sensors that recognize change and adjust the stimulus delivered is important.[34] The advantage of the adaptiveness of closed-loop neuromodulation is based on the iso-response method that consists of the determination of the characteristics of the stimulus response of a neural circuit to elicit a reliably similar neural response.[34,35] SCS sensors monitor the ECAPs, which represent recruitment of fibers in the dorsal column, which is then used to adapt the therapeutic range of stimulation and adjust stimulation in an individualized manner.[28,34]

It is important to notice that although the device has its own intrinsic characteristics to determine the current to close the system loop, like monitoring ECAPs, the user can also play an important role. The information to close the loop can also involve the SCS user turning the device on and off or adjusting the parameters on the fly to better manage the symptoms and to give the user a better sense of control of the device.

In order for these systems to work effectively, it is important that biomarkers translated into a signal that is recognized by a device's sensor inform the system of an accurate and representative dynamic state of the target.[34] The use of closed-loop systems through spinal cord stimulators aims to fulfill this condition with recent demonstrated superior outcome measures compared with open-loop systems.[21]

BASIC COMPONENTS OF A CLOSED-LOOP NEUROMODULATION SYSTEM
Sensors

There are different types of sensors, but those used in closed-loop neuromodulation to measure ECAPs consist of conductive elements placed in the epidural space, potentially being used for sensing and delivering therapy. The Evoke system (Saluda Medical, Sydney, Australia) is the first SCS system to use sensors to measure in vivo neural activity and provide real-time activation of the spinal cord and modulation of neural activity. The Evoke system uses 1 or 2 12-contact leads placed in the epidural space.[30,34]

Acquisition System

The acquisition system can be seen in a simplified way as an equalizer of signals recorded by the sensors. It is responsible for preparing the signal to be used by the processing unit. The acquisition system is responsible for the signal digitalization with good accuracy, rate, and bit-rate resolution through the analog-to-digital converter. The system can also contain bioamplifiers in case the signal output from the sensors needs to be amplified and used to suppress artifact. The acquisition system is a component present in closed-loop stimulators, and can communicate with the processing unit, which usually is within the same physical unit as the acquisition system.[34]

Processing Unit

The processing unit is a computer unit responsible for analyzing the input, comparing it with preprogrammed expectations and physiologic conditions, and calculating and coordinating the output signals to optimize the stimulation settings in the therapeutic window of stimulation. After stimulation, the processing unit algorithm evaluates the preceding interventions, and compares the actual to the desired response to the neurostimulation, calculating the response error. Based on this gap between what was expected versus what was delivered, the computer adjusts the next intervention. In the Evoke system, the programmer communicates with the processing unit to set up the device parameters and the therapeutic window, through a clinical interface and a transceiver.[34,36]

Output Device

The output device is the one that delivers the stimulation that will trigger action potentials, in this case aiming to activate large Aβ dorsal column fibers preferentially. The sensors for the signal input system typically also deliver stimulation.[34,36]

SUITABLE BIOMARKERS

The ECAP is the biomarker unit used to close the loop in spinal cord stimulator systems, although different closed-loop systems use different biomarkers. The neurochemical field of study is broad, and most of the research around new devices consist of the concentration of neurotransmitters such as serotonin, glutamate, and dopamine, or ions such as sodium (Na^+), potassium (K^+), calcium (Ca^{2+}), chloride (Cl^-), or hydrogen (H^+).[37] Different from closed-loop SCS already discussed, chemical biomarkers require biochemical sensors. However, independent of the physical process related to the biomarker measurements, a sensor's output is still an electrical potential evaluated in real time by an acquisition system. These characteristics make chemical biomarkers potentially time efficient for closed-loop neuromodulation and promising alternatives for the future.[34]

WEARABLE AND WIRELESS TECHNOLOGY

Wearables are devices worn in close contact with the targeted region of interest. Applications of wearable sensors allow monitoring of physiologic and biochemical data.[39] With wireless technology, wearables have been used as an input and output unit of neuromodulation and as a wireless communication unit.

Wearables and wireless technology have become more popular in recent years with the popularization of smartphones and increased use of telemedicine, accelerated by the COVID-19 pandemic.[38–40] There are multiple advantages of this promising technology. Having the control units adjacent to the target area, instead of implanted, eliminates the need for multiple replacement surgeries, and consequently the accompanying surgical complications. Another advantage is the ability to monitor and program patients remotely. This is an important feature considering that a great majority of the population lives in rural areas, greatly benefitting by reprogramming without a physically present clinical appointment through wireless direct monitoring and connection with wearable devices. The Evoke system for example, has a pocket console that allows the patient to control therapy and actively monitors stimulator battery status and other elements of the system.[36,41,42]

Although there are multiple advantages with wearables, some challenges exist. The type of connection used by these devices includes Wifi technology, Bluetooth technology, or Zigbee, which can lead to possible interaction with other wireless devices and exposure to electrical or magnetic fields affecting these devices. In addition, the safety of these devices needs to be evaluated cautiously. They are autonomous units being remotely controlled, so the control unit needs to periodically evaluated. Because data are stored in a cloud platform, the possibility of cyberattacks exists.[41,43–45]

There are a few examples of wearable sensors used in closed-loop systems on the market in different neuroscience areas like Parkinson, epilepsy, multiple sclerosis, stroke rehabilitation, and other areas like cardiology and sleep medicine.[38,43,46–51] There are few studies evaluating the impact of wearables on pain management. Davergne and colleagues and Lee and colleagues conducted a meta-analysis assessing the functionality of wearables with regard to tracking activity and providing the user with feedback to evaluate the impact on physical activity; however, given the heterogenous sample, no robust conclusions could be derived.[52,53]

The use of wearables to mediate closed-loop stimulators is promising, and recent studies have been testing wearable models to analyze their efficiency in comparison with wired devices. One of the main issues when evaluating wireless devices as a part of a closed-loop system is the reliability of the communication, and consequently the impact on the device performance. Andreu and colleagues list 5 challenges that need to be overcome by wireless devices for closed-loop neuromodulation compared with wired units: avoidance of collision, optimization of bandwidth occupation, determinism, bounded time latencies for robust control, and safety against frame losses.[41]

In 2019, the US Food and Drug Administration cleared the Freedom SCS Stimwave system as "an adjunct to other modes of therapy used in a multidisciplinary approach for chronic, intractable pain of the trunk and/or lower limbs, including unilateral or bilateral pain."[54] This device is the first passive, electrode-selectable, wireless, microsize stimulator platform for pain management. The device is placed through a 14G needle, adjacent to the target, and uses sensors and high-frequency energy transmission to create the energy field responsible to modulate pain signals at the peripheral nerves and spinal cord. Clinical performance data did demonstrate noninferiority in pain relief at the 6-month follow-up when compared with traditional SCS.[54,55]

SUMMARY

Closed-loop spinal cord stimulators and wearable technology that can be used as a component of the closed-loop system or independently to track and measure bio-signals are promising. ECAPs are the biosignal used for closed-loop neurostimulator systems currently available, but there are new biomarkers being evaluated. Studies have demonstrated the superiority of closed-loop systems in pain management compared with traditional open-loop SCSs. Long-term effects on patient quality of life and functional outcomes still need to be determined. Wearables are promising technology that still need to overcome challenges related to interactions with external devices, and data protection concerns.

DISCLOSURE OF FUNDING

None.

CONFLICT OF INTEREST

None.

REFERENCES

1. Melnikova I. Pain market. Nat Rev Drug Discov 2010;9(8):589.
2. Rao PP, Mohamed T. Current and emerging "at-site" pain medications: a review. J pain Res 2011;4:279.
3. Dissanayake D, Dissanayake D. The physiology of pain: an update and review of clinical relevance. J Ceylon Coll Physicians 2015;46:19–23.
4. Lee GI, Neumeister MW. Pain: pathways and physiology. Clin Plast Surg 2020;47(2):173–80.
5. Hall JE, Hall ME. Guyton and Hall textbook of medical physiology e-Book. Vancouver: Elsevier Health Sciences; 2020.
6. Yam MF, Loh YC, Tan CS, et al. General pathways of pain sensation and the major neurotransmitters involved in pain regulation. Int J Mol Sci 2018;19(8).
7. Melzack R, Wall PD. Pain mechanisms: a new theory. Science 1965;150(3699):971–9.
8. Sdrulla AD, Guan Y, Raja SN. Spinal cord stimulation: clinical efficacy and potential mechanisms. Pain Pract 2018;18(8):1048–67.
9. Sweet WH, Wepsic JG. Treatment of chronic pain by stimulation of fibers of primary afferent neuron. Trans Am Neurol Assoc 1968;93:103–7.
10. Shealy CN, Mortimer JT, Hagfors NR. Dorsal column electroanalgesia. J Neurosurg 1970;32(5):560–4.
11. Nashold BS Jr, Friedman H. Dorsal column stimulation for control of pain. Preliminary report on 30 patients. J Neurosurg 1972;36(5):590–7.
12. Long DM, Erickson D, Campbell J, et al. Electrical stimulation of the spinal cord and peripheral nerves for pain control. A 10-year experience. Appl Neurophysiol 1981;44(4):207–17.
13. Doly S, Fischer J, Brisorgueil MJ, et al. Pre-and post-synaptic localization of the 5-HT7 receptor in rat dorsal spinal cord: immunocytochemical evidence. J Comp Neurol 2005;490(3):256–69.
14. Bardin L. The complex role of serotonin and 5-HT receptors in chronic pain. Behav Pharmacol 2011;22(5 and 6):390–404.
15. Holsheimer J, Struijk JJ. How do geometric factors influence epidural spinal cord stimulation? A quantitative analysis by computer modeling. Stereotact Funct Neurosurg 1991;56(4):234–49.
16. Schultz DM, Webster L, Kosek P, et al. Sensor-driven position-adaptive spinal cord stimulation for chronic pain. Pain Physician 2012;15(1):1–12.
17. Holsheimer J. Principles of neurostimulation. 15, Chapter 3. 2003.
18. Abejon D, Feler CA. Is impedance a parameter to be taken into account in spinal cord stimulation? Pain Physician 2007;10(4):533–40.
19. Barolat G. Epidural spinal cord stimulation: anatomical and electrical properties of the intraspinal structures relevant to spinal cord stimulation and clinical correlations. Neuromodulation 1998;1(2):63–71.
20. Mekhail N, Levy RM, Deer TR, et al. Long-term safety and efficacy of closed-loop spinal cord stimulation to treat chronic back and leg pain (Evoke): a double-blind, randomised, controlled trial. Lancet Neurol 2020;19(2):123–34.
21. Russo M, Brooker C, Cousins MJ, et al. Sustained long-term outcomes with closed-loop spinal cord stimulation: 12-month results of the prospective, multicenter, open-label Avalon study. Neurosurgery 2020;87(4):e485–95.
22. Little S, Pogosyan A, Neal S, et al. Adaptive deep brain stimulation in advanced Parkinson disease. Ann Neurol 2013;74(3):449–57.
23. Rosin B, Slovik M, Mitelman R, et al. Closed-loop deep brain stimulation is superior in ameliorating parkinsonism. Neuron 2011;72(2):370–84.
24. Parker J, Karantonis D, Single P. Hypothesis for the mechanism of action of ECAP-controlled closed-loop systems for spinal cord stimulation. Healthc Technology Lett 2020;7(3):76–80.
25. Parker JL, Karantonis DM, Single PS, et al. Compound action potentials recorded in the human spinal cord during neurostimulation for pain relief. Pain 2012;153(3):593–601.
26. Parker JL, Karantonis DM, Single PS, et al. Electrically evoked compound action potentials recorded from the sheep spinal cord. Neuromodulation 2013;16(4):295–303.
27. Rosen S, Parker J, Obradovic M. Randomized double-blind crossover study examining the safety and effectiveness of closed-loop control in spinal cord stimulation. Paper presented at: North American Neuromodulation Society 19th Annual Meeting. December 10–13, 2015, Las Vegas, NV.
28. Russo M, Cousins MJ, Brooker C, et al. Effective relief of pain and associated symptoms with closed-loop spinal cord stimulation system: preliminary results of the Avalon study. Neuromodulation 2018;21(1):38–47.
29. Brooker C, Russo M, Cousins MJ, et al. ECAP-controlled closed-loop spinal cord stimulation efficacy and opioid reduction over 24-months: final

results of the prospective, multicenter, open-label avalon study. Pain Pract 2021;21(6):680–91.

30. Maher C, Littlewood C. Unanswered questions from the Evoke trial. Lancet Neurol 2020;19(5):380.

31. Knotkova H, Hamani C, Sivanesan E, et al. Neuromodulation for chronic pain. Lancet 2021; 397(10289):2111–24.

32. Xu FL, Hao MZ, Xu SQ, et al. Development of a closed-loop system for tremor suppression in patients with Parkinson's disease. Annu Int Conf IEEE Eng Med Biol Soc 2016;2016:1782–5.

33. te Dorsthorst M, van Balken M, Heesakkers J. Tibial nerve stimulation in the treatment of overactive bladder syndrome: technical features of latest applications. Curr Opin Urol 2020;30(4).

34. Zanos S. Closed-loop neuromodulation in physiological and translational research. Cold Spring Harb Perspect Med 2019;9(11).

35. Gollisch T, Herz AV. The iso-response method: measuring neuronal stimulus integration with closed-loop experiments. Front Neural Circuits 2012;6:104.

36. Medical S. Evoke SCS system clinical manual. Sydney, Australia. 2017.

37. Mirza KB, Golden CT, Nikolic K, et al. Closed-loop implantable therapeutic neuromodulation systems based on neurochemical monitoring. Front Neurosci 2019;13:808.

38. Leroux A, Rzasa-Lynn R, Crainiceanu C, et al. Wearable devices: current status and opportunities in pain assessment and management. Digital Biomarkers 2021;5(1):89–102.

39. Mouchtouris N, Lavergne P, Montenegro TS, et al. Telemedicine in neurosurgery: lessons learned and transformation of care during the COVID-19 pandemic. World Neurosurg 2020;140:e387–94.

40. Franco D, Montenegro T, Gonzalez GA, et al. Telemedicine for the spine surgeon in the age of COVID-19: multicenter experiences of feasibility and implementation strategies. Glob Spine J 2020. 2192568220932168.

41. Andreu D, Sijobert B, Toussaint M, et al. Wireless electrical stimulators and sensors network for closed loop control in rehabilitation. Front Neurosci 2020; 14:117.

42. Health UDo, Services H. Healthcare disparities in rural areas: selected findings from the 2004 national health care disparities report. US Department of Health and Human Services, Agency for Healthcare Research and Quality. 2004.

43. Patel S, Park H, Bonato P, et al. A review of wearable sensors and systems with application in rehabilitation. J neuroengineering Rehabil 2012;9(1):1–17.

44. Groeneveld SA, Jongejan N, de Winter B, et al. Hacking into a pacemaker; risks of smart healthcare devices. Ned Tijdschr Geneeskd 2019;163.

45. Piwek L, Ellis DA, Andrews S, et al. The rise of consumer health wearables: promises and barriers. Plos Med 2016;13(2):e1001953.

46. Morgan C, Rolinski M, McNaney R, et al. Systematic review looking at the use of technology to measure free-living symptom and activity outcomes in Parkinson's disease in the home or a home-like environment. J Parkinson's Dis 2020;10(2):429–54.

47. Salimzadeh Z, Damanabi S, Kalankesh LR, et al. Mobile applications for multiple sclerosis: a focus on self-management. Acta Informatica Med 2019; 27(1):12.

48. Johansson D, Ohlsson F, Krýsl D, et al. Tonic-clonic seizure detection using accelerometry-based wearable sensors: a prospective, video-EEG controlled study. Seizure 2019;65:48–54.

49. Lee J-Y, Kwon S, Kim W-S, et al. Feasibility, reliability, and validity of using accelerometers to measure physical activities of patients with stroke during inpatient rehabilitation. PloS one 2018;13(12): e0209607.

50. Dagher L, Shi H, Zhao Y, et al. Wearables in cardiology: here to stay. Heart Rhythm 2020;17(5):889–95.

51. Pulantara IW, Parmanto B, Germain A. Development of a just-in-time adaptive mHealth intervention for insomnia: usability study. JMIR Hum Factors 2018; 5(2):e8905.

52. Davergne T, Pallot A, Dechartres A, et al. Use of wearable activity trackers to improve physical activity behavior in patients with rheumatic and musculoskeletal diseases: a systematic review and meta-analysis. Arthritis Care Res 2019;71(6):758–67.

53. Li LC, Feehan LM, Xie H, et al. Efficacy of a physical activity counseling program with use of a wearable tracker in people with inflammatory arthritis: a randomized controlled trial. Arthritis Care Res 2020; 72(12):1755–65.

54. FDA/CEDR resources page. Available at: https:// www.fda.gov/medical-devices/device-approvals-denials-and-clearances. Accessed October, 9, 2021.

55. Stimwave T. Freedom spinal cord stimulator clinical manual. Fort Lauderdale. 2015.

The Role of Intrathecal Pumps in Nonmalignant Pain

Elizabeth E. Ginalis, MD[a], Saim Ali, BA[b], Antonios Mammis, MD[b],*

KEYWORDS

- Central nervous system • Intrathecal therapy • Morphine • Neurosurgery • Pain • Ziconotide

KEY POINTS

- Intrathecal therapy allows for efficient medication dosage in patients with chronic pain who have failed conservative pain management options.
- Appropriate patient selection is essential before intrathecal pump insertion.
- More randomized control trials are essential to guide updated guidelines on the intrathecal therapy in the setting of nonmalignant chronic pain.

INTRODUCTION

According to the CDC, 1 in 5 U.S. adults experience chronic pain.[1] Chronic pain is associated with anxiety, depression, and decreased quality of life. As chronic pain continues to be one of the most common reasons for patients to seek medical care, the understanding and advancement of both medical and surgical treatment options is essential.[2,3]

Since Bier's 1898 cocainization of the spinal cord, a multitude of researchers have studied the intrathecal space as a target for drug delivery.[4] Intrathecal therapies allow patients to utilize lower doses of medications as this administration route bypasses the blood–brain barrier and consequently allows for direct delivery into the cerebrospinal fluid. This, in turn, leads to an increase in analgesic efficacy while decreasing systemic side effects common in oral delivery.[5] In the 1970s, as the World Health Organization (WHO) focused on the treatment of cancer pain, the use of intrathecal therapies emerged as an effective technique. After clinical studies, such as that published by Onofrio and colleagues in 1981, helped support the efficacy of implantable pumps for intrathecal drug delivery, intrathecal therapy came into use for chronic and nonmalignant pain syndromes.[6] With the advent of programmable pumps and more advanced dose modulation techniques, the utilization of implanted pumps for the treatment of chronic pain has increased in recent years.[7]

MEDICATION OPTIONS

While multiple drugs have shown efficacy for intrathecal use, the U.S. Food and Drug Administration (FDA) has currently approved three medications for intrathecal administration: morphine, baclofen, and ziconotide.[7] Morphine and ziconotide are commonly prescribed to treat chronic pain, and baclofen is mainly used to treat spasticity.[8] The intrathecal route allows these drugs to circumvent first-pass metabolism and other biological complexities. This allows patients to be treated with a fraction of the dose that would be taken orally.

Morphine

The clinical value of opiates has been studied and put into practice for thousands of years, mainly in the form of opium. Synonymous with early Middle

[a] Department of Neurological Surgery, Rutgers-New Jersey Medical School, 90 Bergen Street, Newark, NJ 07101, USA; [b] Department of Neurological Surgery, New York University Grossman School of Medicine, 1530 Front Street, Suite 400, East Meadow, NY 11554, USA
* Corresponding author. 1530 Front Street, Suite 400, East Meadow, NY 11554.
E-mail address: antonios.mammis@nyulangone.org

Neurosurg Clin N Am 33 (2022) 305–309
https://doi.org/10.1016/j.nec.2022.02.007
1042-3680/22/

Eastern medicine, morphine has been the center of cultural and political conflicts. First isolated from opium in 1805 by Serturner and colleagues and synthesized by Gates and Tschudi in 1956, morphine has been used in the treatment of general pain. However, widespread understanding of its mechanism was not fully understood until demonstrations of mu and other opioid receptors in the 1970s.[9]

Morphine is an opioid analgesic acting as an agonist for mu-, delta-, and kappa-opioid G-protein-linked receptors. The activation of opioid receptors results in a downstream cascade resulting in analgesia through a reduction of nociceptive transmission.[10] Of the opioids, morphine is the only one approved for intrathecal use. Numerous studies have proven morphine's efficacy in treating chronic and nonmalignant pain.[11,12] With robust evidence, morphine remains an effective drug that is commonly used to treat patients with chronic pain. One of its unique properties compared with other opioids is its hydrophilic character, which allows it to spread further following intrathecal administration and consequently increase the area of analgesia. However, as the dose increases, side effects tend to limit the amount that can be taken orally.[13] Intrathecal morphine administration allows targeted delivery of the drug to the dorsal horn of the spinal cord, the location of mu and other opioid receptors.[14]

In a prospective study, Grider and colleagues evaluated low-dose (microdose) intrathecal opioid therapy for treating patients with nonmalignant pain. A total of 58 patients treated with a low dose (fewer than 350 μg per day of morphine equivalent) of intrathecal morphine were found to have sustained analgesic relief and lower pain over the 36-month study period. The average preimplantation visual analog scale (VAS) score was 7.8. After subsequent follow-ups, the average VAS score among the patients was measured at 4.4, 4.8, 5.1, and 4.6 at time points of 6 months, 12 months, 24 months, and 36 months after implantation, respectively. Consistently throughout the study period, VAS scores showed a statistically significant reduction when compared with the preimplantation baseline.[15] Thus, intrathecal medication administration is not only effective, but lasting.

The side effects of oral opioids have been well documented. Systemic effects nausea, anxiety, anorexia, urinary retention, constipation, and pruritus. High doses of intrathecal morphine can cause hyperalgesia, allodynia, and myoclonia.[16] Long-term use can result in reduced libido, impotence, amenorrhea, hypogonadism, and cortisol deficiency.[16] As with all opioids, one of the most dangerous adverse effects is respiratory depression, which can result from rostral distribution of morphine to the ventral medulla. Oral opioid use should be closely monitored due to its high addiction and abuse risk. Tolerance may also develop during long-term therapy, consequently requiring increasing doses over time. Patients should also be counseled on identifying symptoms of withdrawal, including agitation, diarrhea, hyperthermia, and palpitations. Intrathecal therapy may provide a unique advantage to oral opioid use as its dose amount is a fraction of the size of oral prescriptions.[4,17] This results in a reduction in side effects with intrathecal morphine therapy compared with oral therapy and has also shown to decrease the dosage of oral therapy.

Ziconotide

Ziconotide is a nonopioid analgesic that acts as an antagonist to N-type calcium channels, which play a role in neural signal transmission. Ziconotide is a complex synthetic peptide that works by blocking N-type calcium channels. The nociceptive effect of ziconotide is hypothesized to stem from the blocking of neurotransmission in the spinal cord.[17]

Wallace and colleagues conducted a double-blind, placebo-controlled, randomized trial to study the efficacy of intrathecal ziconotide for nonmalignant pain in patients whereby traditional treatments failed. After recording baseline visual analog scale of pain intensity (VASPI) scores, patients on both the ziconotide and control treatment were observed in an in-patient setting over a 6-day period. After this period, VASPI scores of the ziconotide group had reduced by 31.2% from the baseline, compared with a 6.0% reduction in the placebo group. Moreover, after the treatment period, 43.8% of patients in the ziconotide group experienced moderate or better pain relief, and 8.9% expressed complete pain relief. In the placebo group, 73.3% of patients expressed no relief or worsening pain.[18] Other clinical studies have shown similar descriptions of the strong analgesic effect of intrathecal ziconotide. Rauck and colleagues conducted a two-arm, randomized trial to study the efficacy and safety of intrathecal ziconotide. After a 1-week stabilization period to ween patients from current opioid treatments, participants were randomized to placebo or ziconotide. The patients were monitored for 3 weeks and were evaluated on a weekly basis. The percentage improvement of mean VASPI scores was 14.7% for the treatment group and 7.2% in the control group.[19] This difference was statistically significant.

Due to the strong addictive effects of opiates, ziconotide provides a nonopiate analgesic option that maintains efficacy up to 12 months without inducing tolerance or withdrawal.[17] However, ziconotide has a narrow therapeutic window that results in several neurologic side effects, particularly vestibular symptoms from inhibiting N-type calcium channels in the granular cell layer of the cerebellum.[16] Milder side effects include dizziness, nausea, vomiting, nystagmus, and diarrhea. More serious side effects such as cognitive impairment, abnormal gait, urinary retention, psychosis, depression, and creatine kinase elevations may also be associated with ziconotide use.[16] Slower titration and dose modulation can remedy side effects. However, treatment should be discontinued in the setting of more serious side effects.[2] Unfortunately, there is a high risk of side effects during intrathecal therapy which, along with high cost, limits its clinical utility.

DISCUSSION

Although evidence suggests that intrathecal therapy can be a useful method for treating patients with nonmalignant pain, appropriate patient selection and involvement of a multidisciplinary team is essential. Patients with chronic pain are likely to have already gone through extensive patient-driven and medical professional-instructed treatments. At this point, patients need to undergo a personalized treatment regimen that includes evaluation with a pain specialist and neurosurgeon. As an invasive treatment, intrathecal therapy is often the last resort for patients.

Clinical Outcomes

While the evidence for intrathecal medication administration for cancer-related pain has been extensively studied, there is less literature for nonmalignant pain syndromes. To date, studies have shown intrathecal drug administration via implantable pump is safe and effective in reducing pain. In a systematic review by Hayek and colleagues, the long-term efficacy of intrathecal therapy for noncancer pain was examined. They found limited to moderate evidence for the use of intrathecal therapy for nonmalignant pain, with a USPSTF grade of Level II-3. They comment that there is evidence for the use of this technique in patients with noncancer pain, with some inherent limitations.[20] Another study found significant improvement in pain assessment that resulted in greater functional activity following intrathecal pump insertion. Patients' quality of life, activity, and relationships all improved, and the majority were able to return to their professional activities.[21] Similarly, another study found a 27% improvement in the Oswestry Disability Index following intrathecal pump insertion compared with only 12% in the control group receiving convention therapy. Interestingly, their cost analysis showed fewer cumulative costs over the 5-year study period in the pump group and the high initial cost of equipment and surgery was recovered after 28 months.[22]

Indications

Appropriate patient selection and adequate counseling before intrathecal pump insertion are imperative. Patient are considered for intrathecal therapy after failing several conservative treatments and/or experiencing untreatable side effects of opioids. Patients must have no psychological contraindications or cognitive disorders. Additional criteria may include a clear diagnosis, life expectancy greater than 3 months, and a strong social support system. Lastly, patients must have a positive response during the trial period and any other pathology with a surgical indication should be ruled out.

In the setting of nonmalignant pain, intrathecal pump implantation can be an option for patients with nociceptive pain, neuropathic pain, or mixed. Indications include failed back surgery syndrome (FBSS), complex regional pain syndrome (CRPS) type I, neuropathic pain, peripheral neuropathy, spinal stenosis, spinal cord injury, chronic compression fractures, visceral pain, chronic pancreatitis, and postherpetic neuralgia. The FDA states that intrathecal therapy is suitable for patients with intractable pain in the case whereby traditional treatments have failed.[2] [o] The Polyanalgesic Consensus Conference identified multiple indications for treatment by intrathecal therapy, including FBSS, CRPS, axial neck or back pain in patients who are not surgical candidates, abdominal/pelvic pain, extremity pain, trunk pain due to postherpetic neuralgia or post-thoracotomy syndromes, cancer pain, and analgesic efficacy with systemic opioid delivery complicated by intolerable side effects.[23–25] In general, patients with neuropathic pain and localized pain are strong candidates for intrathecal therapy.

Due to its invasive nature, intrathecal therapy is contraindicated for patients with significant medical comorbidities who are not surgical candidates, allergy to intrathecal medications, psychiatric conditions, and spinal infection or sepsis, and patients on anticoagulation that cannot be held perioperatively.[7] Patients with nonlocal pain are less likely to have success from intrathecal therapy.[26]

Trialing

Trialing is necessary before surgical implantation of an intrathecal pump. The goal of trialing is to assess patient response to intrathecal treatment and accurately determine initial dosage needs.[2] With nonmalignant pain, careful titration is needed to establish correct dosing that allows for proper analgesic effect while also limiting the side effects of opiates and pain-relief medications. Trials can be conducted with a bolus injection via lumbar puncture or by placing an intrathecal catheter for either continuous or bolus intrathecal infusion. The patient's pain is self-reported using a VAS score, and the patient is closely monitored for any side effects. Patients are initially started on a low dose that is then titrated up until greater than 50% pain relief without side effects is achieved. Dosage estimations can be calculated using ratio conversions from oral or intravenous treatment.[27] Previous literature has shown that dividing by 12 to 300 for daily oral medication dosing should be a starting point for estimating daily intrathecal dosage. However, standardized techniques are not clearly defined. Post-trial, patients should be monitored by medical staff to ensure patient safety, as all opioid treatments come with risk. Vital signs should be continually measured and naloxone, an opioid antagonist, should be readily available.[4]

Surgical Technique and Considerations

Generally, the patient is placed in the left lateral decubitus position. With fluoroscopy, the intrathecal catheter is inserted into the lower lumbar intrathecal space either percutaneously or using a small incision over the L3-4 or L4-5 level. The catheter tip is then positioned several levels cranially to minimize catheter pullout. The catheter is then secured to the fascial layer using an anchor to reduce displacement. A subcutaneous pocket is then created in the abdominal wall. The catheter is next tunneled in the subcutaneous space to this pocket. The pump is filled with medication, connected to the catheter, and ultimately inserted into a previously created pocket. The tubing should be coiled underneath the pump to prevent inadvertent puncture during future reservoir refill. The pump is programmed accordingly with the daily dose and flow rate. The patient is observed perioperatively and monitored closely for signs of overdose.

Complications

All patients should be counseled regarding complications related to intrathecal therapy. Side effects of the analgesic medication itself are described previously. Hardware-related complications are not uncommon. These include catheter or pump malfunction, catheter dislocation, leakage of catheter, infection, meningitis, seroma, and catheter-associated inflammatory mass.[16] Perioperative complications include bleeding at the insertion site, postdural puncture headaches, cerebrospinal fluid leakage, and epidural hematoma.

SUMMARY

Intrathecal delivery of pain management medications marks a significant step in the treatment of chronic pain. When compared with oral delivery of analgesics, intrathecal therapy has shown to be efficient with few side effects.[19] However, further research, specifically in the form of randomized control trials, is needed to strengthen the evidence for intrathecal therapy. Currently, intrathecal therapy in the setting of nonmalignant pain is often the last resort for these patients. Updated guidelines by experts in the field on the consensus of intrathecal treatment are needed.

CLINICS CARE POINTS

Pearls:

1. Intrathecal therapy delivers analgesic medication directly to the central nervous system, circumventing first-pass metabolism and acting directly on key receptors.

2. Intrathecal pumps allow for precise titration of medication without patient involvement. Dosage can be accurately and efficiently controlled by a medical professional.

Pitfalls:

1. Intrathecal therapy is an invasive procedure, especially when compared with traditional treatment routes such as oral delivery.

2. Hardware-related and medication-related complications can arise, including granuloma formation, infection, and drug overdose.

DISCLOSURE

The authors have nothing to disclose.

REFERENCE

1. Dahlhamer J, Lucas J, Zelaya C, et al. Prevalence of chronic pain and high-impact chronic pain among adults — United States, 2016. MMWR Morb Mortal Wkly Rep 2018;67:1001–6. https://doi.org/10.15585/mmwr.mm6736a2.

2. Deer TR, Pope JE, Hanes MC, et al. Intrathecal therapy for chronic pain: a review of morphine and ziconotide as firstline options. Pain Med 2019;20(4):784–98.

3. Schappert SM, Burt CW. Ambulatory care visits to physician offices, hospital outpatient departments, and emergency departments: United States, 2001–02. National Center for Health Statistics. Vital Health Stat 2006;13(159).

4. Belverud S, Mogilner A, Schulder M. Intrathecal pumps. Neurotherapeutics 2008;5(1):114–22.

5. Bhatia G, Lau ME, Koury KM, et al. Intrathecal drug delivery (ITDD) systems for cancer pain. F1000Res 2013;2:96.

6. Onofrio BM, Yaksh TL, Arnold PG. Continuous low-dose intrathecal morphine administration in the treatment of chronic pain of malignant origin. Mayo Clin Proc. 981;56(8):516–20.

7. Bottros MM, Christo PJ. Current perspectives on intrathecal drug delivery. J Pain Res 2014;7:615–26.

8. Medical Advisory Secretariat. Intrathecal baclofen pump for spasticity: an evidence-based analysis. Ont Health Technol Assess Ser 2005;5(7):1–93.

9. Pasternak GW, Pan YX. Mu opioids and their receptors: evolution of a concept. Pharmacol Rev 2013;65(4):1257–317.

10. Bull FA, Baptista-Hon DT, Lambert JJ, et al. Morphine activation of mu opioid receptors causes disinhibition of neurons in the ventral tegmental area mediated by β-arrestin2 and c-Src. Sci Rep 2017;7:9969. https://doi.org/10.1038/s41598-017-10360-8.

11. Moulin DE, Iezzi A, Amireh R, et al. Randomised trial of oral morphine for chronic non-cancer pain. Lancet 1996;347(8995):143–7.

12. Busse JW, Wang L, Kamaleldin M, et al. Opioids for chronic noncancer pain: a systematic review and meta-analysis. JAMA 2018;320(23):2448–60.

13. Gupta S, Atcheson R. Opioid and chronic non-cancer pain. J Anaesthesiol Clin Pharmacol 2013;29(1):6–12.

14. Kerchner GA, Zhuo M. Presynaptic suppression of dorsal horn inhibitory transmission by mu-opioid receptors. J Neurophysiol 2002;88(1):520–2.

15. Grider JS, Etscheidt MA, Harned ME, et al. Trialing and maintenance dosing using a low-dose intrathecal opioid method for chronic nonmalignant pain: a prospective 36-month study. Neuromodulation 2016;19(2):206–19.

16. Ver Donck A, Vranken JH, Puylaert M, et al. Intrathecal drug administration in chronic pain syndromes. Pain Pract 2014;14(5):461–76.

17. McGivern JG. Ziconotide: a review of its pharmacology and use in the treatment of pain. Neuropsychiatr Dis Treat 2007;3(1):69–85.

18. Wallace MS, Charapata SG, Fisher R, et al. Intrathecal ziconotide in the treatment of chronic nonmalignant pain: a randomized, double-blind, placebo-controlled clinical trial. Neuromodulation 2006;9(2):75–86.

19. Rauck RL, Wallace MS, Leong MS, et al. A randomized, double-blind, placebo-controlled study of intrathecal ziconotide in adults with severe chronic pain. J Pain Symptom Manage 2006;31(5):393–406.

20. Hayek SM. Intrathecal therapy for cancer and non-cancerpain. Pain Physician 2011;14(3):219–48. https://doi.org/10.36076/ppj.2011/14/219.

21. Duse G, Davià G, White PF. Improvement in psychosocial outcomes in chronic pain patients receiving intrathecal morphine infusions. Anesth Analg 2009;109(6):1981–6.

22. Kumar K, Hunter G, Demeria DD. Treatment of chronic pain by using intrathecal drug therapy compared with conventional pain therapies: a cost-effectiveness analysis. J Neurosurg 2002;97(4):803–10.

23. Deer TR, Hayek SM, Pope JE, et al. The Polyanalgesic Consensus Conference (PACC): Recommendations for Trialing of Intrathecal Drug Delivery Infusion Therapy. Neuromodulation 2017;20(2):133–54.

24. Deer TR, Pope JE, Hayek SM, et al. The Polyanalgesic Consensus Conference (PACC): Recommendations on Intrathecal Drug Infusion Systems Best Practices and Guidelines. Neuromodulation 2017;20(2):96–132.

25. Deer TR, Pope JE, Hayek SM, et al. The Polyanalgesic Consensus Conference (PACC): Recommendations for Intrathecal Drug Delivery: Guidance for Improving Safety and Mitigating Risks. Neuromodulation 2017;20(2):155–76.

26. The polyanalgesic consensus conference (PACC): recommendations on intrathecal drug infusion systems best practices and guidelines. Neuromodulation 2017;20(4):405–6.

27. Gerber HR. Intrathecal morphine for chronic benign pain. Best Pract Res Clin Anaesthesiol 2003;17(3):429–42. https://doi.org/10.1016/S1521-6896(03)00014-4. Available at: https://www.sciencedirect.com/science/article/pii/S1521689603000144.

Deep Brain Stimulation for Chronic Pain

Alexander Alamri, MBBS, BSc, FHEA, MRCS*,
Erlick A.C. Pereira, MA(Camb), DM(Oxf), FRCS(NeuroSurg)

KEYWORDS

- Deep brain stimulation • Chronic pain • Ventral posterior thalamus
- Periaqueductal gray/periventricular gray • Anterior cingulate cortex

KEY POINTS

- Key targets include the periaqueductal gray, periventricular gray, ventral posterior thalamus, and anterior cingulate cortex.
- Several decades of case series evidence exist, with varying operative techniques and clinical outcomes.
- Further trials that are randomised, double-blinded, and placebo controlled will help to define the true benefit of this treatment.

BACKGROUND

Prior to the 1960s, the mainstay of treating neurologic disorders was targeted surgical lesioning of specific cortical and subcortical brain structures. The first report of human cortical stimulation was described by Bartholow in 1874 following the Fritsch and Hitzig experiments of 1870, where electrical stimulation of animal brains and the motor cortex showed localized electrical excitability.[1]

The introduction of stereotaxy by neurosurgeons, such as Victor Horsley in the early twentieth century, meant that the safe and accurate targeting of deeper subcortical structures became possible in a reproducible manner.[2] Lesioning of the globus pallidus or thalamus became a relatively more widespread surgical intervention, which was guided by intraoperative stimulation of subcortical structures. Deep brain stimulation (DBS) truly gained momentum in the mid-1960s due to the theoretic paradigm shift initiated by Melzack and Wall's[3] gate theory and advances in stimulator technology. Gate theory allowed for the development of implantable peripheral nerve stimulators[4] and then spinal cord stimulation (SCS)[5] into a commercially available, permanently implantable device.[6,7] Since then, DBS has provided dramatic clinical benefits for movement disorders, such as Parkinson disease and essential tremor, as well as psychiatric disorders, such as obsessive-compulsive disorder (OCD).[8–13]

There has been burgeoning interest in the use of DBS for chronic pain refractory to medical treatment. The various indications include phantom limb pain,[14–18] brachial plexus injury,[17–20] post-stroke pain,[15–17,20,21] facial pain,[15,22,23] spinal injuries, failed back surgery syndrome,[15–17,24] and headaches.[23,25,26]

MECHANISMS OF ACTION

There currently is no accepted definition of the mechanism of action of DBS on underlying interconnected neural networks. At the neuronal level, electrical stimulation causes a depolarization event, but this does not explain the global network effect of stimulation. High-frequency stimulation has been shown to suppress or inhibit the activity of target neurons, likening the effect of DBS to a reversible lesion. From insights revealed by basal ganglia microelectrode recordings and DBS for movement disorders, altered rhythmic activity in

Neurosciences Research Centre, Molecular and Clinical Sciences Institute, St George's University of London, London, United Kingdom
* Corresponding author.
E-mail address: aalamri@sgul.ac.uk

Neurosurg Clin N Am 33 (2022) 311–321
https://doi.org/10.1016/j.nec.2022.02.013

the ventral posterior lateral (VPL) and ventral posterior medial (VPM) thalamus and the periventricular gray (PVG)/periaqueductal gray (PAG) neurons results in the pathophysiology of central pain.[27–29] At either target, DBS at lower frequencies ($\leq$50 Hz) is analgesic and higher frequencies (>70 Hz) hyperalgesic,[30–32] indicating a dynamic model whereby synchronous oscillations in discrete neuronal populations centrally modulate chronic pain perception. Therefore, DBS may be exerting its effect either by disrupting high-frequency synchronous oscillations, or by "boosting" diminished low-frequency oscillations in the thalamic and reticular components of a reticulo-thalamic-corticofugal pain neuromatrix.

Several studies in animals and humans have demonstrated the PAG and thalamus as crucial structures of pain perception and involved in chronic pain pathologies.[33–42] Ventral posterior (VP) thalamic stimulation may work through non-opioid mechanisms and can offer some relief in central pain.[43] In contrast, it has been hypothesized that PAG DBS induces opioidergic or autonomic mechanisms in pain processing.[44–46]

PAIN PATHWAYS

The PAG and ventrobasal thalamus are structures important to pain perception and the pathophysiology of chronic pain syndromes. Evidence for this has been posited through radiological, anatomic, and electrophysiologic evidence in humans and animals.[33,35,37,38,40–42,47,48] The subtleties of hierarchical position and behavioral function of individual brain structures, whether sensory-discriminative, attentional, motivational-affective, or hedonic, are much debated. The prevailing paradigm, however, is toward a pain neuromatrix also involving spinal cord, posterior hypothalamus, amygdala, and neocortical structures, including somatosensory, insular, anterior cingulate, and prefrontal cortex.[3,49] The predominant brain structures that are involved in pain signaling following a noxious stimulus include the anterior cingulate cortex (ACC), insula, thalamus, lentiform nuclei, cerebellum and somatosensory cortex. These pathways have been described and attributed to a medial and a lateral pain system, both of which have been shown to be modulated by stimulation.[50,51]

The lateral system comprises VPL, VPM, and VP inferior nuclei of the thalamus as well as the lateral spinothalamic tract. As a result, the lateral system is responsible for the sensory-discriminative role in pain perception.

The medial system plays a role in emotional, cognitive, somatosensory and sympathetic autonomic processing. Anatomically, this is made up of the rostral to dorsal ACC and the anterior insular cortex.

ANATOMICAL TARGETS

Targets for DBS as a treatment of chronic pain have been described variably in the literature. Several distinct regions have been targeted historically, including the septal region,[52,53] thalamic VPL and VPM nuclei,[14–17,20,54–59] PVG and PAG,[15–17,21,57,59–61] internal capsule,[59,61] posterior hypothalamus,[23,26,62] nucleus accumbens,[21] and ACC.[19,63]

A central tenet of DBS surgery is that the anatomic target acts as a basis for the intended placement for the stimulating electrode, but that final target selection requires some form of physiologic mapping or clinical assessment. For example, although identification and initial entry into sensory thalamus may be based on anatomic data, it is essential to define the thalamic homunculus physiologically and place the electrode accordingly. The two methodologies most employed to achieve electrophysiological confirmation are stimulation or recording of the neural activity.

The Sensory Nuclei of the Thalamus (Ventral Posterior Lateral and Ventral Posterior Medial)

Ablative surgery in the 1960s provided inroads into the characterization of the VPL and VPM with regard to their role in pain.[64] As reported in large case series of DBS for chronic pain, sensory thalamic stimulation has been used with varying effectiveness in several chronic pain syndromes,[24,65] with the VPM particularly targeted in facial pain.[66] Thalamic targets are 10 mm to 13 mm posterior to the midcommissural point. Depending on the pain site, the best location can be from 5 mm inferior to 2 mm superior the intercommissural line. The VPM, targeted for face pain only, is found between the wall of the third ventricle and the internal capsule. The VPL is targeted 2 mm to 3 mm medial to the internal capsule for the arm pain, and 1 mm to 2 mm for the leg area. The stimulation induces a pleasant paresthesia in the painful area.

Anterior Cingulate Cortex

The *neuromatrix theory of pain* is based on cognitive-evaluative, sensory-discriminative, and motivational-affective components. The ACC is an anatomic hub for these affective components and, as such, has proved to be a target for the treatment of chronic pain.[67–70] The ACC itself is part of the cingulate gyrus and consists of Brodmann areas 24, 25, 32, and 33. Neuromodulation of the ACC and surrounding areas has been performed to treat other disorders, primarily psychiatric and affective ones. The subcallosal cingulate was targeted for OCD and depression,[71,72] and DBS of the anterior limb of internal capsule (ALIC) was US Food and Drug Administration approved for OCD. Furthermore, in central poststroke pain, the stimulation of the ALIC/nucleus accumbens has been described as a potential target for the affective component.[21]

The ACC lies on the medial surface of the frontal lobe and extends from the premotor cortex before turning rostrally with the genu of the corpus callosum and then quarterly, ventral to the callosum. It has various roles and functions within various networks, including emotion, motivation, and determining value.[67,73–80] Surgical cingulotomy traditionally has been performed for the treatment of medically refractory cancer pain, neuropathic pain, lower back pain, reflex sympathetic dystrophy, upper abdominal, and lower thoracic pain.[81–88] Ballantine and colleagues'[75] 1967 study on 35 patients suffering from pain due to terminal cancer showed good relief following cingulotomy. Patients reported that it was not the ability to localize a noxious stimulus or the intensity of it that had been modulated but rather the affective response to it. Patients typically reported that they were no longer "bothered" by the pain. The rostral ACC (Cg24) recently was targeted for DBS (**Fig. 1**) based on functional neuroimaging demonstrating its activation as well as evidence from cancer pain lesioning.[63,84,89,90]

Periaqueductal Gray and Periventricular Gray

Initially, the PVG and PAG were identified as targets for DBS in animal research. In the first animal studies, rodents underwent surgical procedures while concurrently having PAG stimulation. This was the only analgesic modality required for pain control.[91,92] These findings were translated to humans later on and widely used by several functional neurosurgeons.[22,60,93] Evidence supporting VPL/VPM and VP thalamic nuclei and adjacent structures as putative targets for DBS came from ablative surgery,[64,94–96] leading Hosobuchi and colleagues[97] to treat anesthesia dolorosa with VPM thalamic DBS.

The PVG is surrounded by the medial lemniscus laterally, superior colliculus posteriorly, and red nucleus anteriorly. The DBS electrode is placed 2 mm to 3 mm lateral to the third ventricle at the level of the posterior commissure (PC). When these areas are stimulated, the pain is substituted by a

sensation of warmth or analgesia. Stimulation of the PVG also induces some modulation of autonomic functions.[98–100]

The PAG is located circumferentially around the aqueduct of Sylvius extending from the PC down to the locus coeruleus (LC) caudally. It has a vital role in the descending modulation of pain perception and as such is a key target for treating chronic pain.[101] The PAG also is responsible for the modulation of sympathetic responses, pain, and learned aversive behaviors. Nociceptive signals that ascend from the dorsal horns via the spinothalamic, and spinal bulbar pathways then ascend via the PAG to the medial thalamus. The predominant descending pathways include the LC and the ventral medial medulla (VMM). The PAG-LC pathway has an inhibitory effect on nociception in the dorsal horn, acting via noradrenaline. The PAG-VMM pathway depends on serotonin as a major nociceptive modulator endogenously. This pathway exerts its effects by inhibiting neurotransmission to C-fiber afferents.

In cases of the PVG or PAG targets, stimulation induces feelings of warmth or well-being when the proper target is stimulated. Thresholds for macrostimulation should be 0.5 V to 3 V. Test stimulation using the DBS electrode confirms placement accuracy and checks for potential untoward side effects. Levels of stimulation higher than 1 V to 3 V may recruit more distant structures and lead to erroneous clinical judgments by the surgeon, such as if side effects occur resulting in a false-negative clinical correlation. The PAG target is found at a point 2 mm to 3 mm lateral to the third ventricle at the level of the PC, 10 mm posterior to the midcommissural point (**Table 1**). Important anatomic boundaries in the midbrain include the medial lemniscus laterally, superior colliculus inferoposteriorly, and red nucleus inferoanteriorly. The sensory thalamus is bordered by the centromedian and parafascicular nuclei medially; internal capsule laterally, thalamic fasciculus, zona incerta, and subthalamic nucleus inferiorly; thalamic nucleus ventralis intermedius anteriorly; and pulvinar thalamic nucleus posteriorly. The rostral ACC target area Cg24 is 20 mm to 25 mm posterior to the anterior horns of the lateral ventricles with electrode tips abutting the corpus callosum.

PATIENT SELECTION

As part of the initial clinical evaluation, it is important to ensure that a patient's pain is medically intractable. The screening process should be initiated by a pain physician with experience in the management of chronic pain syndromes. In some instances, psychological assessment also

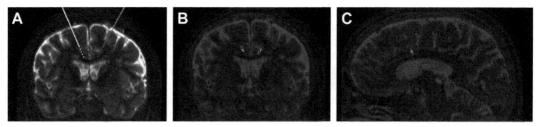

Fig. 1. Views of bilateral electrodes in the ACC. (*A*) Preoperative trajectory planning. (*B*) Coronal view. (*C*) Sagittal view on postoperative fused MRI/CT images.

should take place, together with a detailed history of the nature, location, and onset of the pain. A psychological assessment ascertains whether there is potential for pain relief and to assess the presence and severity of potential underlying psychiatric disorders. This can be a relative or absolute contraindication for implantation of any neuromodulation device. Alternative surgical therapies to DBS, such as SCS, intrathecal medications, motor cortex stimulation, and ablative surgery, always can be considered. In all cases of pain management, it is important to correct underlying anatomic pathophysiologic mechanisms that induce or perpetuate pain. For example, DBS should not be used as a first-line treatment of spondylotic disease, but it may be appropriate for patients who have failed conservative or first-line surgical therapies for failed back surgery syndromes, such as SCS. When DBS appears to be a reasonable option for a specific pain syndrome, it is important to explain the risks and benefits of surgery. Surgical complications for DBS are low but include hemorrhage causing disability (0.3%) and death (0.1%). Other complications include perioperative or delayed infection (up to 6 months) and skin erosion over the implant. Reported benefits in the literature vary greatly,[17,102–107] but up to two-thirds of patients can experience a 50% or greater symptomatic gain in the long term.[102] Loss of stimulation efficacy over time (tolerance) is a well-described phenomenon in neuromodulation for pain and it may or sometimes may not respond to changes of stimulation parameters.

OPERATIVE CONSIDERATIONS

The degree of DBS implantation accuracy for optimal therapeutic outcome remains poorly

Table 1
Anatomical targets, stereotactic coordinates, and their local structures in deep brain stimulation for pain

Anatomic Target	Location	Stereotactic Coordinates	Adjacent Structures
VPL	1–3 mm medial (leg 1–2 mm, arm 2–3 mm) to internal capsule at level of PC	10–13 mm posterior to midcommissural point, 14–18 mm lateral, 2–5 mm vertical	Internal capsule laterally; centromedian and parafascicular thalamic nuclei medially; thalamic fasciculus, zona incerta, subthalamic nucleus inferiorly; thalamic nucleus ventralis intermedius anteriorly; pulvinar thalamic nucleus posteriorly
VPM	Midway between wall of third ventricle and internal capsule, at level of PC		
PVG/PAG	PVG 2–3 mm lateral to wall of third ventricle, at level of PC. PAG deeper adjacent to the aqueduct of Sylvius	PVG 10 mm posterior to midcommissural point, 2–3 mm lateral, 0 mm vertical	PAG: medial lemniscus laterally; superior colliculus inferoposteriorly; red nucleus inferoanteriorly

defined in chronic pain. In general, however, in DBS surgery the difference between the planned and actual electrode position should not exceed 2 mm unless moved by awake testing.[108] After the setup of a reference system for target localization, the patient undergoes magnetic resonance imaging (MRI) or computed tomography (CT). Then, the target and anterior commissure (AC)-PC line are delineated. The patient then is brought to the operating room and placed in some form of head fixation for frame-based systems. For most of the commonly used targets, the initial target coordinates can be defined with respect to the AC-PC plane. These coordinates should deliver the mapping electrode into the presumed physiologic target. From that point on, electrophysiologic definition of the target via macroelectrode stimulation in the awake patient will better refine the ultimate resting place for the electrode. Burr holes are placed approximately 3 cm from the midline on or anterior to the coronal suture. The exact location of the hole should be defined explicitly with a presurgical trajectory. Draping systems should allow for interaction with the patient and yet maintain a sterile field. To minimize cerebrospinal fluid leakage, the dura and underlying arachnoid are penetrated with the twist drill, or, if a burr hole is used, they are rapidly opened and fibrin glue is applied to obliterate the hole. This is important to prevent cerebrospinal fluid loss and entrance of air, which can jointly distort intracranial structures because of brain shift and postoperative pneumocephalus. The treatment electrode should be introduced with great care to ensure that it reaches the desired target locus and then tested physiologically. The electrode should be functionally tested using macrostimulation to assess location and adverse effects. The homuncular organization differs between thalamic and PVG/PAG targets.[109,110] In the ventroposterior thalamus the homuncular head is medial, with the feet lateral, implying a mediolateral somatotopy.[105] A more rostro-caudally inverted sensory homunculus in PVG/PAG has been confirmed objectively by our human macroelectrode recordings of somatosensory evoked potentials.[46] Initially, bipolar stimulation between 5 Hz and 50 Hz can be trialed, with a pulse-width of 100 ms to 450 ms and an amplitude of 0.1 V to 3 V. Stimulation-induced paresthesia in the targeted area of pain indicates ideal electrode placement in the sensory thalamus. If both criteria are met, the electrode may be anchored using a variety of available systems, including locking caps or miniplates. and the pulse generator implanted and connected. Clinical sequelae to be aware of in VPL/VPM DBS include pyramidal signs, suggesting capsular involvement.

In PAG/PVG, adverse effects include oscillopia from involvement of the superior colliculus and facial paresthesia due to stimulation of the medial lemniscus. With regard to the ACC, intraoperative and postoperative stimulation might not cause a clinical effect for days to weeks afterward, making intraoperative stimulation testing redundant. Finally, de novo stimulation-induced epilepsy has been reported in a small cohort of patients undergoing ACC stimulation, overcome by cycling stimulatin.[111]

DISCUSSION

Worldwide, since the first brain stimulation studies in the 1950s,[22,52,53,59,61,112,113] only a few groups have published larger case series on DBS for chronic pain.[14–17,19,20,57,62]

There have been two multicenter trials of DBS for pain were performed to seek US Food and Drug Administration approval. The first trial in 1976 enrolled 196 patients and the second trial in 1990 enrolled 50 patients.[51] The criterion to satisfy the trials was that at least half of patients should report 50% pain relief at 1 year postoperatively, which was not achieved in either trial, with the second trial closing early due to slow enrollment and poor efficacy. There have been 22 case studies and series reported in the literature to date, which have been predominantly open-label and non-randomized, with the exceptions of Marchand and colleagues[20] and Fontaine and colleagues.[114] Seventeen series and studies (200 patients) targeted VPM/VPL or PAG matter, ACC (24 patients), VS/ALIC (10 patients), centromedian and parafascicular nuclei of the thalamus (3 patients), and posterior limb of the internal capsule (3 patients). Results from the Oxford group showed that 59/85 of patients retained their electrodes 6 months after surgery, and 39/59 of those operated on described a sustained global improvement.[17,115]

Finally, even when DBS is truly efficacious in some patients, tolerance may manifest after several years. It could be overcome by slight changes in stimulation settings or by interrupting the stimulation periodically. Further technological advancements, such as adaptive stimulation, might allow patients to experience reduced tolerance and better efficacy of treatment.

SUMMARY

DBS for pain has been shown effective in several case series using three main targets: PAG/PVG, VPM/VPL, and ACC. Ensuring appropriate patient selection and rigorous planning is vital. The next steps require clinical trials to demonstrate the efficacy of DBS to treat intractable chronic pain. Because DBS can be switched on and off, randomized controlled trials with smaller patient populations can be achieved.

CLINICS CARE POINTS

- Key targets include the PAG, PVG, VP thalamus, and ACC.
- Several decades of case series evidence exist, with varying operative techniques and clinical outcomes.
- Further trials that are randomized, double-blinded, and placebo-controlled will help to define the true benefit of this treatment.

DISCLOSURE

The authors report no external funding or conflicts of interest.

REFERENCES

1. Fritsch G, Hitzig E. Über die elektrische Erregbarkeit des Grosshirn [On the Electrical Excitability of the Cerebrum]. Archive für Anatomie, Physiologie und wissenschaftliche Medicin. 1870;37:300–32.
2. Pereira EAC, Green AL, Nandi D, et al. Stereotactic neurosurgery in the United Kingdom: The hundred years from Horsley to Hariz. Neurosurgery 2008; 63(3):594–606.
3. Melzack R, Wall PD. Pain mechanisms: a new theory. Science 1965;150(699):971–9. Available at: http://www.ncbi.nlm.nih.gov/entrez/query.fcgi?cmd=Retrieve&db=PubMed&dopt=Citation&list_uids=5320816.
4. Sweet WH, Wepsic JG. Treatment of chronic pain by stimulation of fibers of primary afferent neuron. Trans Am Neurol Assoc 1968;93:103–7. Available at: http://www.ncbi.nlm.nih.gov/entrez/query.fcgi?cmd=Retrieve&db=PubMed&dopt=Citation&list_uids=5304599.
5. Shealy CN, Mortimer JT, Reswick JB. Electrical inhibition of pain by stimulation of the dorsal columns: preliminary clinical report. Anesth Analg 1967;46(4):489–91. Available at: http://www.ncbi.nlm.nih.gov/entrez/query.fcgi?cmd=Retrieve&db=PubMed&dopt=Citation&list_uids=4952225.
6. Mullett K. Electrical brain stimulation for the control of chronic pain. Med Instrum 1978;12(2):88–91.

Available at: http://www.ncbi.nlm.nih.gov/entrez/query.fcgi?cmd=Retrieve&db=PubMed&dopt=Citation&list_uids=308150.
7. Mullett K. State of the art in neurostimulation. Pacing Clin Electrophysiol 1987;10(1 Pt 2):162–75. Available at: http://www.ncbi.nlm.nih.gov/entrez/query.fcgi?cmd=Retrieve&db=PubMed&dopt=Citation&list_uids=2436175.
8. Chabardes S, Isnard S, Castrioto A, et al. Surgical implantation of STN-DBS leads using intraoperative MRI guidance: technique, accuracy, and clinical benefit at 1-year follow-up. Acta Neurochir 2015. https://doi.org/10.1007/s00701-015-2361-4.
9. Deep Brain Stimulation for Parkinson's Disease Study G. Deep-brain stimulation of the subthalamic nucleus or the pars interna of the globus pallidus in Parkinson's disease. N Engl J Med 2001;345(13): 956–63, 11575287.
10. Aziz TZ, Bain PG. Deep brain stimulation in Parkinson's disease. J Neurol Neurosurg Psychiatr 1999; 67(3):281, 0010449546.
11. Montgomery EB Jr. Deep brain stimulation reduces symptoms of Parkinson disease. Cleve Clin J Med 1999;66(1):9–11, 0009926625.
12. Yianni J, Aziz T. Globus pallidus internus deep brain stimulation for dystonic conditions. Neurol Sci 2003;24:S277–80.
13. Bittar RG, Yianni J, Wang S, et al. Deep brain stimulation for generalised dystonia and spasmodic torticollis. J Clin Neurosci 2005;12(1):12–6, 15639404.
14. Yamamoto T, Katayama Y, Obuchi T, et al. Thalamic sensory relay nucleus stimulation for the treatment of peripheral deafferentation pain. Stereotact Funct Neurosurg 2006;84(4):180–3. Available at: http://www.ncbi.nlm.nih.gov/entrez/query.fcgi?cmd=Retrieve&db=PubMed&dopt=Citation&list_uids=16905881.
15. Hamani C, Schwalb JM, Rezai AR, et al. Deep brain stimulation for chronic neuropathic pain: long-term outcome and the incidence of insertional effect. Pain 2006;125(1–2):188–96. Available at: http://www.ncbi.nlm.nih.gov/entrez/query.fcgi?cmd=Retrieve&db=PubMed&dopt=Citation&list_uids=16797842.
16. Rasche D, Foethke D, Gliemroth J, et al. [Deep brain stimulation in the posterior hypothalamus for chronic cluster headache Case report and review of the literature. 2006. Available at: http://www.ncbi.nlm.nih.gov/entrez/query.fcgi?cmd=Retrieve&db=PubMed&dopt=Citation&list_uids=16404629.
17. Boccard SG, Pereira EA, Moir L, et al. Long-term Outcomes of Deep Brain Stimulation for Neuropathic Pain. Neurosurgery 2013;72(2):221–31.

Available at: http://www.ncbi.nlm.nih.gov/entrez/query.fcgi?cmd=Retrieve&db=PubMed&dopt=Citation&list_uids=23149975.

18. Pereira EA, Aziz TZ. Reincarnating the oxford cingulectomy in the epoch of stereotaxy and resurrecting lesions in the era of deep brain stimulation. Stereotact Funct Neurosurg 2013;91(4):262–3.

19. Boccard SG, Pereira EA, Moir L, et al. Deep brain stimulation of the anterior cingulate cortex: targeting the affective component of chronic pain. Neuroreport 2014;25(2):83–8.

20. Marchand S, Kupers RC, Bushnell MC, et al. Analgesic and placebo effects of thalamic stimulation. Pain 2003;105(3):481–8. Available at: http://www.ncbi.nlm.nih.gov/entrez/query.fcgi?cmd=Retrieve&db=PubMed&dopt=Citation&list_uids=14527708.

21. Mallory GW, Abulseoud O, Hwang SC, et al. The nucleus accumbens as a potential target for central poststroke pain. Mayo Clin Proc 2012;87(10):1025–31.

22. Hosobuchi Y, Wemmer J. Disulfiram inhibition of development of tolerance to analgesia induced by central gray stimulation in humans. Eur J Pharmacol 1977;43(4):385–7. Available at: http://www.ncbi.nlm.nih.gov/entrez/query.fcgi?cmd=Retrieve&db=PubMed&dopt=Citation&list_uids=880983.

23. Franzini A, Ferroli P, Leone M, et al. Stimulation of the posterior hypothalamus for treatment of chronic intractable cluster headaches: first reported series. Neurosurgery 2003;52(5):1095–9.

24. Pereira EA, Boccard SG, Linhares P, et al. Thalamic deep brain stimulation relieves neuropathic pain after amputation or brachial plexus avulsion. Neurosurg Focus 2013;35(3):1–11.

25. Bartsch A, Samorezov S, Benzel E, et al. Validation of an "Intelligent Mouthguard" Single Event Head Impact Dosimeter. Stapp Car Crash J 2014;58:1–27. Available at: http://sfxeu05.hosted.exlibrisgroup.com/44RCS?sid=OVID:medline&id=pmid:26192948&id=doi:&issn=1532-8546&isbn=&volume=58&issue=&spage=1&pages=1-27&date=2014&title=Stapp+Car+Crash+Journal&atitle=Validation+of+an+%22Intelligent+Mouthguard%22+Single+Event+Head.

26. Nguyen JP, Lefaucheur JP, Decq P, et al. Chronic motor cortex stimulation in the treatment of central and neuropathic pain. Correlations between clinical, electrophysiological and anatomical data. Pain 1999;82(3):245–51, 10488675.

27. Brown P. Oscillatory nature of human basal ganglia activity: Relationship to the pathophysiology of Parkinson's disease. Movement Disord 2003;18(4):357–63.

28. Engel AK, Moll CK, Fried I, et al. Invasive recordings from the human brain: clinical insights and beyond. Nat Rev Neurosci 2005;6(1):35–47. Available at: http://www.ncbi.nlm.nih.gov/entrez/query.fcgi?cmd=Retrieve&db=PubMed&dopt=Citation&list_uids=15611725.

29. Hutchison WD, Dostrovsky JO, Walters JR, et al. Neuronal oscillations in the basal ganglia and movement disorders: evidence from whole animal and human recordings. J Neurosci 2004;24(42):9240–3. Available at: http://www.ncbi.nlm.nih.gov/entrez/query.fcgi?cmd=Retrieve&db=PubMed&dopt=Citation&list_uids=15496658.

30. Nandi D, Aziz TZ. Deep brain stimulation in the management of neuropathic pain and multiple sclerosis tremor. J Clin Neurophysiol 2004;21(1):31–9. Available at: http://www.ncbi.nlm.nih.gov/entrez/query.fcgi?cmd=Retrieve&db=PubMed&dopt=Citation&list_uids=15097292.

31. Bittar RG, Burn SC, Bain PG, et al. Deep brain stimulation for movement disorders and pain. J Clin Neurosci 2005;12(4):457–63, 15925782.

32. Pereira EA, Moir L, McIntyre C, et al. Deep brain stimulation for central post-stroke pain – relating outcomes and stimulation parameters in 21 patients. Acta Neurochir 2008;150(9):968.

33. Romanelli P, Heit G. Patient-controlled deep brain stimulation can overcome analgesic tolerance. Stereotact Funct Neurosurg 2004;82(2–3):77–9. Available at: http://www.ncbi.nlm.nih.gov/entrez/query.fcgi?cmd=Retrieve&db=PubMed&dopt=Citation&list_uids=15305078.

34. Romanelli P, Esposito V. The functional anatomy of neuropathic pain. Neurosurg Clin N Am 2004;15(3):257–68. Available at: http://www.ncbi.nlm.nih.gov/entrez/query.fcgi?cmd=Retrieve&db=PubMed&dopt=Citation&list_uids=15246335.

35. Peyron R. Parietal and cingulate processes in central pain. A combined positron emission tomography (PET) and functional magnetic resonance imaging (fMRI) study of an unusual case. Pain 2000;84:77–87.

36. Tracey I. Functional connectivity and pain: how effectively connected is your brain? Pain 2005;116(3):173–4. Available at: http://www.ncbi.nlm.nih.gov/entrez/query.fcgi?cmd=Retrieve&db=PubMed&dopt=Citation&list_uids=15982816.

37. Sewards T v, Sewards MA. The medial pain system: neural representations of the motivational aspect of pain. Brain Res Bull 2002;59(3):163–80. Available at: http://www.ncbi.nlm.nih.gov/entrez/

query.fcgi?
cmd=Retrieve&db=PubMed&dopt=Citation&list_
uids=12431746.

38. Gauriau C, Bernard JF. Pain pathways and para-brachial circuits in the rat. Exp Physiol 2002;87(2): 251–8. Available at: http://www.ncbi.nlm.nih.gov/entrez/query.fcgi?
cmd=Retrieve&db=PubMed&dopt=Citation&list_
uids=11856971.

39. Willis WD, Westlund KN. Neuroanatomy of the pain system and of the pathways that modulate pain. J Clin Neurophysiol 1997;14(1):2–31. Available at: http://www.ncbi.nlm.nih.gov/entrez/query.fcgi?
cmd=Retrieve&db=PubMed&dopt=Citation&list_
uids=9013357.

40. Behbehani MM. Functional characteristics of the midbrain periaqueductal gray. Prog Neurobiol 1995;46(6):575–605, 8545545.

41. Craig AD. Pain mechanisms: labeled lines versus convergence in central processing. Annu Rev Neurosci 2003;26:1–30. Available at: http://www.ncbi.nlm.nih.gov/entrez/query.fcgi?
cmd=Retrieve&db=PubMed&dopt=Citation&list_
uids=12651967.

42. Kupers R, Kehlet H. Brain imaging of clinical pain states: a critical review and strategies for future studies. Lancet Neurol 2006;5(12):1033–44. Available at: http://www.ncbi.nlm.nih.gov/entrez/query.fcgi?
cmd=Retrieve&db=PubMed&dopt=Citation&list_
uids=17110284.

43. Date I, Felten SY, Felten DL. Cografts of adrenal medulla with peripheral nerve enhance the surviv-ability of transplanted adrenal chromaffin cells and recovery of the host nigrostriatal dopaminergic system in MPTP-treated young adult mice. Brain Res 1990;537(1–2):33–9, 0001982243.

44. Akil H, Richardson DE, Hughes J, et al. Enkephalin-like material elevated in ventricular cerebrospinal fluid of pain patients after analgetic focal stimula-tion. Science 1978;201(4354):463–5. Available at: http://www.ncbi.nlm.nih.gov/entrez/query.fcgi?
cmd=Retrieve&db=PubMed&dopt=Citation&list_
uids=663668.

45. Akil H, Mayer DJ, Liebeskind JC. Antagonism of stimulation-produced analgesia by naloxone, a narcotic antagonist. Science 1976;191(4230): 961–2. Available at: http://www.ncbi.nlm.nih.gov/entrez/query.fcgi?
cmd=Retrieve&db=PubMed&dopt=Citation&list_
uids=1251210.

46. Pereira EA, Wang S, Owen SL, et al. Human peri-ventricular grey somatosensory evoked potentials suggest rostrocaudally inverted somatotopy. Ster-eotact Funct Neurosurg 2013;91(5):290–7.

47. Tracey I. Nociceptive processing in the human brain. Curr Opin Neurobiol 2005;15(4):478–87.

Available at: http://www.ncbi.nlm.nih.gov/entrez/query.fcgi?
cmd=Retrieve&db=PubMed&dopt=Citation&list_
uids=16019203.

48. Willis WD Jr. Pain pathways in the primate. Prog Clin Biol Res 1985;176:117–33. Available at: http://www.ncbi.nlm.nih.gov/entrez/query.fcgi?
cmd=Retrieve&db=PubMed&dopt=Citation&list_
uids=3923492.

49. Loeser JD, Melzack R. Pain: An overview. Lancet 1999;353(9164). https://doi.org/10.1016/S0140-6736(99)01311-2.

50. Volkers R, Giesen E, van der Heiden M, et al. Inva-sive Motor Cortex Stimulation Influences Intracere-bral Structures in Patients With Neuropathic Pain: An Activation Likelihood Estimation Meta-Analysis of Imaging Data. Neuromodulation 2020;23(4). https://doi.org/10.1111/ner.13119.

51. Coffey RJ. Deep brain stimulation for chronic pain: results of two multicenter trials and a structured review. Pain Med (Malden, Mass) 2001;2(3): 183–92.

52. Heath RG. Psychiatry. Annu Rev Med 1954;5: 223–36, 13181376.

53. Gol A. Relief of pain by electrical stimulation of the septal area. J Neurol Sci 1967;5(1):115–20. Avail-able at: http://www.ncbi.nlm.nih.gov/entrez/query.fcgi?
cmd=Retrieve&db=PubMed&dopt=Citation&list_
uids=6061755.

54. Mazars G, Roge R, Mazars Y. [Results of the stimulation of the spinothalamic fasciculus and their bearing on the physiopathology of pain. Rev Prat 1960;103:136–8. Available at: http://www.ncbi.nlm.nih.gov/entrez/query.fcgi?
cmd=Retrieve&db=PubMed&dopt=Citation&list_
uids=13768640.

55. Hosobuchi Y. Motor cortical stimulation for control of central deafferentation pain. Adv Neurol 1993; 63:215–7. Available at: http://www.ncbi.nlm.nih.gov/entrez/query.fcgi?
cmd=Retrieve&db=PubMed&dopt=Citation&list_
uids=8279306.

56. Levy R, Hazrati LN, Herrero MT, et al. Re-evaluation of the functional anatomy of the basal ganglia in normal and Parkinsonian states. Neuroscience 1997;76(2):335–43, 9015319.

57. Kumar K, Toth C, Nath RK. Deep brain stimulation for intractable pain: a 15-year experience. Neuro-surgery 1997;40(4):736–46. Available at: http://www.ncbi.nlm.nih.gov/entrez/query.fcgi?
cmd=Retrieve&db=PubMed&dopt=Citation&list_
uids=9092847.

58. Turnbull IM, Shulman R, Woodhurst WB. Thalamic stimulation for neuropathic pain. J Neurosurg 1980; 52(4):486–93. Available at: http://www.ncbi.nlm.nih.gov/entrez/query.fcgi?

cmd=Retrieve&db=PubMed&dopt=Citation&list_uids=6966326.

59. Young RF, Kroening R, Fulton W, et al. Electrical stimulation of the brain in treatment of chronic pain. Experience over 5 years. J Neurosurg 1985;62(3):389–96. Available at: http://www.ncbi.nlm.nih.gov/entrez/query.fcgi?cmd=Retrieve&db=PubMed&dopt=Citation&list_uids=3871844.

60. Richardson DE Akil H. Pain reduction by electrical brain stimulation in man. Part 2: Chronic self-administration in the periventricular gray matter. J Neurosurg 1977;47(2):184–94. Available at: http://www.ncbi.nlm.nih.gov/entrez/query.fcgi?cmd=Retrieve&db=PubMed&dopt=Citation&list_uids=301558.

61. Levy RM, Lamb S, Adams JE. Treatment of chronic pain by deep brain stimulation: long term follow-up and review of the literature. Neurosurgery 1987;21(6):885–93. Available at: http://www.ncbi.nlm.nih.gov/entrez/query.fcgi?cmd=Retrieve&db=PubMed&dopt=Citation&list_uids=3325851.

62. Fernandez-Gonzalez F, Seijo F, Menendez-Guisasola L, et al. [Stereotactic target identification for neurosurgery of Parkinson disease]. Rev Neurol 1999;28(6):600–8, 0010714346.

63. Spooner J, Yu H, Kao C, et al. Neuromodulation of the cingulum for neuropathic pain after spinal cord injury. Case report. J Neurosurg 2007;107(1):169–72. Available at: http://www.ncbi.nlm.nih.gov/entrez/query.fcgi?cmd=Retrieve&db=PubMed&dopt=Citation&list_uids=17639889.

64. Mark VH, Ervin FR. Role of Thalamotomy in Treatment of Chronic Severe Pain. Postgrad Med 1965;37:563–71. Available at: http://www.ncbi.nlm.nih.gov/entrez/query.fcgi?cmd=Retrieve&db=PubMed&dopt=Citation&list_uids=14285799.

65. Pereira EA, Wang S, Peachey T, et al. Elevated gamma band power in humans receiving naloxone suggests dorsal periaqueductal and periventricular gray deep brain stimulation produced analgesia is opioid mediated. Exp Neurol 2013;239:248–55. Available at: http://www.ncbi.nlm.nih.gov/entrez/query.fcgi?cmd=Retrieve&db=PubMed&dopt=Citation&list_uids=23127542.

66. Hosobuchi Y, Adams JE, Linchitz R. Pain relief by electrical stimulation of the central gray matter in humans and its reversal by naloxone. Science 1977;197(4299):183–6, 301658.

67. Bush G, Luu P, Posner MI. Cognitive and emotional influences in anterior cingulate cortex. Trends Cogn Sci 2000;4(6):215–22. Available at: http://www.ncbi.nlm.nih.gov/entrez/query.fcgi?

cmd=Retrieve&db=PubMed&dopt=Citation&list_uids=10827444.

68. Rainville P, Duncan GH, Price DD, et al. Pain affect encoded in human anterior cingulate but not somatosensory cortex. Science 1997;277(5328):968–71. Available at: http://www.ncbi.nlm.nih.gov/entrez/query.fcgi?cmd=Retrieve&db=PubMed&dopt=Citation&list_uids=9252330.

69. Paus T. Primate anterior cingulate cortex: where motor control, drive and cognition interface. Nat Rev Neurosci 2001;2(6):417–24. Available at: http://www.ncbi.nlm.nih.gov/entrez/query.fcgi?cmd=Retrieve&db=PubMed&dopt=Citation&list_uids=11389475.

70. Lenz FA, Rios M, Zirh A, et al. Painful stimuli evoke potentials recorded over the human anterior cingulate gyrus. J Neurophysiol 1998;79(4):2231–4. Available at: http://www.ncbi.nlm.nih.gov/entrez/query.fcgi?cmd=Retrieve&db=PubMed&dopt=Citation&list_uids=9535984.

71. Lozano AM, Giacobbe P, Hamani C, et al. A multicenter pilot study of subcallosal cingulate area deep brain stimulation for treatment-resistant depression. J Neurosurg 2012;116(2):315–22.

72. Mayberg HS, Lozano AM, Voon V, et al. Deep brain stimulation for treatment-resistant depression. Neuron 2005;45(5):651–60. Available at: http://www.ncbi.nlm.nih.gov/entrez/query.fcgi?cmd=Retrieve&db=PubMed&dopt=Citation&list_uids=15748841.

73. Devinsky O, Morrell MJ, Vogt BA. Contributions of anterior cingulate cortex to behaviour. Brain 1995;118(Pt 1):279–306. Available at: http://www.ncbi.nlm.nih.gov/pubmed/7895011.

74. Sharma T. Abolition of opiate hunger in humans following bilateral anterior cingulotomy. Tex Med 1974;70(10):49–52. Available at: http://www.ncbi.nlm.nih.gov/entrez/query.fcgi?cmd=Retrieve&db=PubMed&dopt=Citation&list_uids=4421555.

75. Ballantine HT Jr, Cassidy WL, Flanagan NB, et al. Stereotaxic anterior cingulotomy for neuropsychiatric illness and intractable pain. J Neurosurg 1967;26(5):488–95. Available at: http://www.ncbi.nlm.nih.gov/entrez/query.fcgi?cmd=Retrieve&db=PubMed&dopt=Citation&list_uids=5337782.

76. Bush G, Vogt BA, Holmes J, et al. Dorsal anterior cingulate cortex: a role in reward-based decision making. Proc Natl Acad Sci U S A 2002;99(1):523–8. Available at: http://www.ncbi.nlm.nih.gov/entrez/query.fcgi?cmd=Retrieve&db=PubMed&dopt=Citation&list_uids=11756669.

77. Williams ZM, Bush G, Rauch SL, et al. Human anterior cingulate neurons and the integration of monetary reward with motor responses. Nat Neurosci 2004;7(12):1370–5. Available at: http://www.ncbi.nlm.nih.gov/entrez/query.fcgi?cmd=Retrieve&db=PubMed&dopt=Citation&list_uids=15558064.

78. Pujol J, Lopez A, Deus J, et al. Anatomical variability of the anterior cingulate gyrus and basic dimensions of human personality. Neuroimage 2002;15(4):847–55. Available at: http://www.ncbi.nlm.nih.gov/entrez/query.fcgi?cmd=Retrieve&db=PubMed&dopt=Citation&list_uids=11906225.

79. Bush G. Dorsal anterior cingulate cortex: a role in reward-based decision-making. Proc Natl Acad Sci USA 2002;99:523–8.

80. Zubieta JK. Regulation of human affective responses by anterior cingulate and limbic [mu]-opioid neurotransmission. Arch Gen Psychiatry 2003;60:1145–53.

81. Ballantine HT, Cosgrove GR, Giriunas IE. Surgical treatment of intractable psychiatric illness and chronic pain by stereotactic cingulotomy. In: Schmidek HH, Sweet WH, editors. Oper Neurosurg Tech Indications, Methods Results 1995;2:1423–30. Saunders.

82. Hassenbusch SJ. Cingulotomy for cancer pain. In: Gildenberg P, Tasker R, editors. Textbook of stereotactic and functional Neurosurgery. McGraw Hill; 1997. p. 1447–51. Available at: http://www.ncbi.nlm.nih.gov/entrez/query.fcgi?cmd=Retrieve&db=PubMed&dopt=Citation&list_uids=2200976.

83. Gonzalzez ER. Treating the brain by cingulotomy. JAMA 1980;244(19):2141–3, 2146-2147. Available at: http://www.ncbi.nlm.nih.gov/entrez/query.fcgi?cmd=Retrieve&db=PubMed&dopt=Citation&list_uids=6775102.

84. Foltz EL, White LEJr. Pain relief by frontal cingulotomy. J Neurosurg 1962;19:89–94.

85. Yen CP, Kung SS, Su YF, et al. Stereotactic bilateral anterior cingulotomy for intractable pain. J Clin Neurosci 2005;12(8):886–90. Available at: http://www.ncbi.nlm.nih.gov/entrez/query.fcgi?cmd=Retrieve&db=PubMed&dopt=Citation&list_uids=16326270.

86. Wilkinson HA, Davidson KM, Davidson RI. Bilateral anterior cingulotomy for chronic noncancer pain. Neurosurgery 1999;45(5):1129–34. Available at: http://www.ncbi.nlm.nih.gov/entrez/query.fcgi?cmd=Retrieve&db=PubMed&dopt=Citation&list_uids=10549929.

87. Pereira EA, Paranathala M, Hyam JA, et al. Anterior cingulotomy improves malignant mesothelioma pain and dyspnoea. Br J Neurosurg 2013. https://doi.org/10.3109/02688697.2013.857006.

88. Mempel E, Dietrich-Rap Z. [Favorable effect of cingulotomy on gastric crisis pain]. Neurol Neurochir Pol 1977;11(5):611–3. Available at: http://www.ncbi.nlm.nih.gov/entrez/query.fcgi?cmd=Retrieve&db=PubMed&dopt=Citation&list_uids=593512.

89. Cosgrove GR, Rauch SL. Stereotactic cingulotomy. Neurosurg Clin N Am 2003;14(2):225–35. Available at: http://www.ncbi.nlm.nih.gov/entrez/query.fcgi?cmd=Retrieve&db=PubMed&dopt=Citation&list_uids=12856490.

90. Viswanathan A, Harsh V, Pereira EA, et al. Cingulotomy for medically refractory cancer pain. Neurosurg Focus 2013;35(3):E1. https://doi.org/10.3171/2013.6.FOCUS13236.

91. Mayer DJ, Wolfle TL, Akil H, et al. Analgesia from electrical stimulation in the brainstem of the rat. Science 1971;174(16):1351–4. Available at: http://www.ncbi.nlm.nih.gov/entrez/query.fcgi?cmd=Retrieve&db=PubMed&dopt=Citation&list_uids=5167502.

92. Reynolds D v. Surgery in the rat during electrical analgesia induced by focal brain stimulation. Science 1969;164(878):444–5. Available at: http://www.ncbi.nlm.nih.gov/entrez/query.fcgi?cmd=Retrieve&db=PubMed&dopt=Citation&list_uids=4887743.

93. Richardson DE Akil H. Long term results of periventricular gray self-stimulation. Neurosurgery 1977;1(2):199–202, 308192.

94. White JC, Sweet WH. Pain and the neurosurgeon. Charles C Thoms; 1969.

95. Ervin FR, Brown CE, Mark VH. Striatal influence on facial pain. Confin Neurol 1966;27(1):75–90. Available at: http://www.ncbi.nlm.nih.gov/entrez/query.fcgi?cmd=Retrieve&db=PubMed&dopt=Citation&list_uids=5955976.

96. Mark VH, Ervin FR, Hackett TP. Clinical aspects of stereotactic thalamotomy in the human. Part I. The treatment of chronic severe pain. Arch Neurol 1960;3:351–67. Available at: http://www.ncbi.nlm.nih.gov/entrez/query.fcgi?cmd=Retrieve&db=PubMed&dopt=Citation&list_uids=13766885.

97. Hosobuchi Y, Adams JE, Rutkin B. Chronic thalamic stimulation for the control of facial anesthesia dolorosa. Arch Neurol 1973;29(3):158–61. Available at: http://www.ncbi.nlm.nih.gov/entrez/query.fcgi?cmd=Retrieve&db=PubMed&dopt=Citation&list_uids=4591720.

98. Green AL, Wang S, Owen SL, et al. Controlling the heart via the brain: a potential new therapy for orthostatic hypotension. Neurosurgery 2006;58(6):1176–83. Available at: http://www.ncbi.nlm.nih.gov/entrez/query.fcgi?

cmd=Retrieve&db=PubMed&dopt=Citation&list_uids=16723897.

99. Pereira EA, Lu G, Wang S, et al. Ventral peri-aqueductal grey stimulation alters heart rate variability in humans with chronic pain. Exp Neurol 2010;223(2):574–81. Available at: http://www.ncbi.nlm.nih.gov/entrez/query.fcgi?cmd=Retrieve&db=PubMed&dopt=Citation&list_uids=20178783.

100. Pereira EA, Wang S, Paterson DJ, et al. Sustained reduction of hypertension by deep brain stimulation. J Clin Neurosci 2010;17(1):124–7. Available at: http://www.ncbi.nlm.nih.gov/entrez/query.fcgi?cmd=Retrieve&db=PubMed&dopt=Citation&list_uids=19664927.

101. Sillery E, Bittar RG, Robson MD, et al. Connectivity of the human periventricular-periaqueductal gray region. J Neurosurg 2005;103(6):1030–4. Available at: http://www.ncbi.nlm.nih.gov/entrez/query.fcgi?cmd=Retrieve&db=PubMed&dopt=Citation&list_uids=16381189.

102. Boccard SGJ, Prangnell SJ, Pycroft L, et al. Long-Term Results of Deep Brain Stimulation of the Anterior Cingulate Cortex for Neuropathic Pain. World Neurosurg 2017;106. https://doi.org/10.1016/j.wneu.2017.06.173.

103. Tasker RR, Vilela Filho O. Deep brain stimulation for neuropathic pain. Stereotact Funct Neurosurg 1995;65(1–4):122–4. Available at: http://www.ncbi.nlm.nih.gov/entrez/query.fcgi?cmd=Retrieve&db=PubMed&dopt=Citation&list_uids=8916340.

104. Ray CD, Burton C v. Deep brain stimulation for severe, chronic pain. Acta Neurochir Suppl (Wien) 1980;30:289–93. Available at: http://www.ncbi.nlm.nih.gov/entrez/query.fcgi?cmd=Retrieve&db=PubMed&dopt=Citation&list_uids=7008523.

105. Bittar RG, Otero S, Carter H, et al. Deep brain stimulation for phantom limb pain. J Clin Neurosci 2005;12(4):399–404. Available at: http://www.ncbi.nlm.nih.gov/entrez/query.fcgi?cmd=Retrieve&db=PubMed&dopt=Citation&list_uids=15925769.

106. Garonzik I, Samdani A, Ohara S, et al. Deep brain stimulation for the control of pain. Epilepsy Behav 2001;2(3 SUPPL. 3). Available at: http://www.scopus.com/scopus/inward/record.url?eid=2-s2.0-23044462989&partner=40&rel=R4.5.0.

107. Levy RM. Deep brain stimulation for the treatment of intractable pain. Neurosurg Clin N Am 2003;14(3):389–399, vi. Available at: http://www.ncbi.nlm.nih.gov/entrez/query.fcgi?cmd=Retrieve&db=PubMed&dopt=Citation&list_uids=14567140.

108. Li Z, Zhang JG, Ye Y, et al. Review on Factors Affecting Targeting Accuracy of Deep Brain Stimulation Electrode Implantation between 2001 and 2015. Stereotactic Funct Neurosurg 2016;94(6):351–62.

109. Ohara S, Lenz FA. Reorganization of somatic sensory function in the human thalamus after stroke. Ann Neurol 2001;50(6):800–3. Available at: http://www.ncbi.nlm.nih.gov/entrez/query.fcgi?cmd=Retrieve&db=PubMed&dopt=Citation&list_uids=11761479.

110. Lenz FA. Painful stimuli evoke potentials recorded over the human anterior cingulate gyrus. J Neurophysiol 1998;79:2231–4.

111. Maslen H, Cheeran B, Pugh J, et al. Unexpected Complications of Novel Deep Brain Stimulation Treatments: Ethical Issues and Clinical Recommendations. Neuromodulation : J Int Neuromodulation Soc 2018;21(2):135–43.

112. Mazars G, Merienne L, Cioloca C. [Treatment of certain types of pain with implantable thalamic stimulators]. Neurochirurgie 1974;20(2):117–24. Available at: http://www.ncbi.nlm.nih.gov/entrez/query.fcgi?cmd=Retrieve&db=PubMed&dopt=Citation&list_uids=4418054.

113. Mundinger F. [New stereotactic treatment of spasmodic torticollis with a brain stimulation system (author's transl)]. Med Klin 1977;72(46):1982–6, 337081.

114. Fontaine D, Lazorthes Y, Mertens P, et al. "Safety and efficacy of deep brain stimulation in refractory cluster headache: a randomized placebo-controlled double-blind trial followed by a 1-year open extension. J Headache Pain 2010;11(1):23–31.

115. Owen SL, Green AL, Stein JF, et al. Deep brain stimulation for the alleviation of post-stroke neuropathic pain. Pain 2006;120(1–2):202–6. Available at: http://www.ncbi.nlm.nih.gov/entrez/query.fcgi?cmd=Retrieve&db=PubMed&dopt=Citation&list_uids=16359796.

What's New in Peripheral Nerve Stimulation

Hart P. Fogel, BA[a], Christopher J. Winfree, MD[b],*

KEYWORDS

- Chronic pain • Craniofacial pain • Facial pain • Neuromodulation • Neurosurgery
- Peripheral nerve stimulation • Postamputation pain • Postoperative pain

KEY POINTS

- Peripheral nerve stimulation (PNS) is a useful treatment option for the management of intractable pain within the sensory territory innervated by a peripheral nerve.
- Procedural and technological innovations including new stimulation modalities, ultrasound-guided percutaneous electrode implantation, and wireless pulse generators render PNS less invasive and disruptive and pave the way for new applications of the technique.
- PNS is effective for the treatment of a variety of pain disorders, including craniofacial pain, postoperative pain, and postamputation pain.
- Although PNS classically targets the sensory portions of the nerves, PNS targeting of motor nerves is becoming increasingly useful for a variety of chronic pain conditions.
- PNS is also emerging as a potentially useful therapy for a variety of non-pain indications.

INTRODUCTION

Peripheral nerve stimulation (PNS) is a neuromodulation technique whereby electrical current is delivered directly to a peripheral nerve by an electrode array placed next to the target nerve. Once stimulation is initiated, pain relief can occur in the territory of the target nerve. It is one of the earliest published forms of neuromodulation, dating back to 1967.[1,2] Although the early implantable systems were primitive, patients often experienced significant pain relief. Subsequent iterations of PNS systems used repurposed spinal cord stimulator devices. Recent advancements have created dedicated PNS devices that are minimally invasive, safe, and prone to fewer device-related complications than the older systems. There is an emerging evidence base supporting the use of PNS in both pain and non–pain-related conditions.

DISCUSSION
Mechanism of Action

PNS was developed following the description of the gate control theory of pain by Melzack and Wall in 1965.[3] This model posits that the stimulation of large diameter non-nociceptive afferent nerve fibers activates interneurons in the dorsal horn of the spinal cord which, in turn, inhibit the propagation of pain signals from small-diameter nociceptive afferent fibers through the spinal cord to the brain. Subsequent studies have elaborated on this explanation, offering additional mechanisms by which PNS may ameliorate pain. The mechanisms at play are likely quite complicated and have yet to be fully elucidated.

Peripherally, PNS reduces the incidence of ectopic action potentials and downregulates neurotransmitters and pro-inflammatory molecules.[4] It may also decrease the concentration of

a Columbia University Vagelos College of Physicians and Surgeons, 35 Fort Washington Avenue, 6D, New York, NY 10032, USA; b Department of Neurological Surgery, Columbia University, 710 West 168th Street, 4th, Floor, New York, NY 10032, USA
* Corresponding author.
E-mail address: cjw12@cumc.columbia.edu

Neurosurg Clin N Am 33 (2022) 323–330
https://doi.org/10.1016/j.nec.2022.02.009

prostaglandins and endorphins that are responsible for increased blood flow in the setting of chronic pain. In a rat model of sciatic nerve damage, PNS improved nerve regeneration and reduced markers of inflammation including calcitonin gene-related peptide expression.[5] Similarly, a study on colitis in rats demonstrated that vagal nerve stimulation and sacral nerve stimulation are both capable of downregulating pro-inflammatory cytokines such as TNF-α, MCP-1, IL-6, and IL-17A and promoting the anti-inflammatory IL-10.[6]

The analgesic effects of PNS can also be attributed to its action on the central nervous system. Stimulation of the greater occipital nerve in a rat model of trigeminal neuropathic pain modulated pathways of gamma-aminobutyric acid and glycine signaling in the spinal cord.[7] Additionally, a study involving a rat bone cancer model found that PNS-mediated upregulation of activity-regulated cytoskeleton-associated protein and downregulation of GluA1 (a type of glutamate receptor) in the dorsal horn of the spinal cord corresponded with a reduction in hyperalgesia and allodynia.[8] Various other investigations have shown that PNS affects the brain too, promoting descending pathways of pain inhibition via the anterior cingulate cortex and the parahippocampal area as well as elevating blood flow to regions including the insular cortex, thalamus, anteroventral insula, and primary somatosensory cortex.[5]

Patient Selection

Candidates for this therapy should generally have pain in a peripheral nerve distribution and have failed pharmacotherapy and, if appropriate, less invasive interventional treatments. They should not have any ongoing infection or coagulopathy. As is true for patients undergoing trials of other forms of neuromodulation, a psychological screening should be completed before the implantation of the electrode system. Candidates should be aware of the minimal procedural risks and be willing and able to participate in the therapy.[9]

Open Lead Placement

Before the development of the new percutaneous PNS systems, PNS electrodes were typically placed following surgical exposure of the target nerve. Once the nerve was exposed, an electrode array was sewn to the nerve and then tunneled with extension wires to an external generator for a trial period, usually lasting several days. If the patient did well, then another surgery was required to discard the extension wire and connect the array to an implantable pulse generator (IPG). If they did not get sufficient pain relief with the trial, then the system was explanted. Although these systems worked reasonably well, they were prone to complications, including migration, lead fracture, nerve entrapment, and nerve injury. They also required 2 open surgical approaches, regardless of whether the patient had success with or failed the therapy. Given the developments described later in discussion, these open systems are infrequently used.

Percutaneous Lead Placement

Percutaneously placed PNS systems are useful for targeting superficial nerves that are not in proximity to vascular or other vulnerable structures. The supraorbital, infraorbital, and occipital nerves are best suited for this approach. These systems usually use existing spinal cord stimulator electrodes and IPGs, although dedicated PNS systems are now available. The trial leads are typically placed using curved needles and small stab incisions. Given the ease of placement, imaging is rarely needed, although fluoroscopy can be helpful in confirming that the leads, once placed, do not migrate during the procedure. The leads are externalized through the skin for the duration of the trial, and subsequently removed and discarded in the office at the end of the trial. Permanent placement is conducted in a similar fashion, except that the leads are anchored using small incisions and tunneled to an IPG located along the chest wall or back.

Trigeminal branch stimulation, most commonly involving the supraorbital and infraorbital nerves, can be an effective treatment of trigeminal neuropathic pain, Type 2 trigeminal neuralgia, trigeminal deafferentation pain, and trigeminal postherpetic neuralgia.[10] A study from 2020 followed 15 patients with refractory facial pain that was idiopathic, posttraumatic, postherpetic or poststroke in origin who received fluoroscopy-guided supraorbital stimulation and/or infraorbital stimulation; on average, they experienced a 74.3% reduction in pain.[11] Another article describes fluoroscopy-guided supraorbital stimulation that provided substantial pain relief to 15 out of 18 patients with herpes zoster ophthalmicus.[12] Beyond its applications for pain management, trigeminal stimulation was recently found to be capable of inducing vasodilation of cerebral vasculature in a rat model of subarachnoid hemorrhage, leading some to propose that it be investigated as a possible treatment of cerebral vasospasm.[13]

Occipital nerve stimulation is an effective treatment of occipital neuralgia,[14] cervicogenic headache, occipital headache, cluster headache, and migraine.[15] One study reported substantial decreases in pain among 60 patients who underwent occipital nerve stimulation for refractory occipital headaches (albeit with a relatively high rate of lead migration and infection).[16] Similarly, in a review of 96 patients with disorders including migraine, cervicogenic headache, cluster headache and neuropathic scalp pain, occipital nerve stimulation and/or supraorbital stimulation provided long-term relief in 57.1% of cases.[17]

Peripheral Nerve Stimulation Waveforms

Historically, PNS has used low-frequency (ie, tonic) stimulation, which causes paresthesias in the distribution of the target nerve. However, alternative waveforms have been developed in recent years. These waveforms are thought to work through different mechanisms of action than tonic stimulation. These newer waveforms also do not produce paresthesias, which is sometimes preferable for patients.[18,19]

High-frequency (10 kHz) stimulation provides stimulus impulses to the nerve so rapidly that the nerve is unable to repolarize after initial firing. This results in nerve blockade. Patients with a variety of craniofacial pain conditions have benefitted from this technique.[20,21] In a trial comparing outcomes in 58 recipients of high-frequency spinal cord stimulation and 11 recipients of high-frequency PNS, the latter group experienced greater decreases in pain and disability as recorded at 3 to 6 months post stimulation.[22] High-frequency stimulation has also been investigated in postamputation pain with some success.[23]

Burst stimulation is another new waveform that can be effective at subperception levels. The stimulation is comprised of a repeating pattern of several high-frequency impulses followed by a pause. The pattern is designed to provoke a response in certain nervous system pathways that respond preferentially to these burst patterns. One pathway of particular interest is the medial pain pathway, which mediates the affective component of pain. Burst stimulation, in addition to reducing actual pain levels through the lateral pain pathway, also reduces the negative emotional effects of the pain, likely by altering activity in the medial pain pathway. Burst stimulation was comparable to low-frequency tonic stimulation in terms of pain reduction in a study following 7 patients suffering from trigeminal neuropathic pain.[24] Additionally, Burst stimulation of the occipital nerve successfully decreased the frequency and severity of headaches in 17 patients with chronic migraine and chronic cluster headache.[25]

Permanent, Percutaneous, Ultrasound-Guided Peripheral Nerve Stimulation Systems

Although percutaneous PNS placement for superficial nerves such as the trigeminal or occipital nerve may be accomplished using palpable landmarks, the implantation of PNS electrode arrays along deeper nerves requires ultrasound guidance to prevent injury to deeper structures. Using a portable ultrasound device, one can visualize lead position in relation to anatomic structures in real-time. This technique was first used over a decade ago in patients with chronic neuropathic pain, enabling the stimulation of the median, radial, ulnar, peroneal, and posterior tibial nerves.[26] Although initial reports describe ultrasound-guided PNS placement using repurposed SCS systems,[27] dedicated PNS systems are now commercially available. These systems use an introducer needle that is advanced toward the target nerve using ultrasound guidance. Once the needle is in position, the electrode is placed along the nerve. The electrode has small tines that limit the risk of lead migration. The electrode is then left under the skin, with the distal end in the subcutaneous space. The distal end receives input from an external pulse generator, which is placed on the skin immediately over the distal end of the electrode. These systems do not require extensive electrode tunneling or an IPG, thus avoiding their associated complications.

One commercially available device is FDA-approved for the treatment of intractable peripheral mononeuropathy and has effectively alleviated pain and ameliorated patient quality of life in randomized clinical trials.[28] Other studies have described percutaneous, ultrasound-guided PNS for chronic pain along almost every named nerve, as well as for complex regional pain syndrome, dermatomal pain, and postamputation pain.[21,29-37] Other systems for IPG-free PNS are in development, including one that uses a small implanted device (1.7 mm³) containing a piezoceramic transducer to convert ultrasound emitted by an external generator into electrical current.[38]

Temporary, Percutaneous, Ultrasound-Guided Peripheral Nerve Stimulation Systems

A growing body of evidence indicates that in certain instances, percutaneous, ultrasound-guided PNS can provide long-term relief of chronic pain even when the stimulation is only applied temporarily (ie, over a period of up to 60 days). The mechanisms underlying long-term analgesia afforded by short-term stimulation are still being explored. One plausible theory is that the focal, robust, non-nociceptive signals transmitted from the periphery to the central nervous system in PNS promote "reconditioning" in the somatosensory cortex, potentially mitigating maladaptive cortical plasticity that may be partly responsible for some intractable pain conditions alongside peripheral and spinal sensitization.[39]

One commercially available system has been used in this manner to address various pain conditions and currently has FDA clearance for chronic pain. The device consists of an external pulse generator connecting to a coil-shaped percutaneous lead that can be removed at the end of the stimulation period. This sort of "open coil" electrode has been shown to be less likely to migrate or cause infection, as its helical structure allows for fibrotic tissue ingrowth that stabilizes the lead and prevents "pistoning" that may introduce bacteria.[40] Additionally, the system is MRI-compatible, even if the lead fractures.[41]

Peripheral Nerve Stimulation for Postamputation Pain

Many patients who undergo limb amputation subsequently experience debilitating pain that may come in 2 forms: residual limb pain localized to the remaining portion of the extremity and phantom limb pain perceived to be affecting the amputated body part. Whereas the former is typically precipitated by peripheral factors such as neuroma formation, the latter is believed to emerge as a result of neuroplastic processes in the central nervous system.[42] In any case, this pain is often poorly mitigated by medication, so clinicians have been exploring new management modalities including PNS.

Most of the literature on stimulation for postamputation pain has focused on the lower extremity; case reports have described substantial pain relief following ultrasound-guided percutaneous PNS (in combination with a perineural nerve block catheter in one instance and targeted muscle reinnervation in another) in patients with either residual limb pain or both residual and phantom limb pain that was resistant to conventional treatment.[43–47] A randomized controlled trial involving 28 traumatic lower extremity amputation patients found that those who received 8 weeks of femoral and sciatic nerve stimulation experienced significantly greater reductions in pain intensity and interference with daily functioning in weeks 1 to 4 than those who received 4 weeks of placebo and then 4 weeks of crossover PNS.[32] Furthermore, 12 months later, the 8-week stimulation group reported decreased pain intensity and depression.[48]

More recently, case reports regarding the upper extremity have been published. One patient with residual and phantom limb pain experienced analgesia after ultrasound-guided percutaneous PNS targeting the radial nerve.[49] Another had phantom limb pain that was alleviated by brachial plexus stimulation.[50]

Peripheral Nerve Stimulation for Acute Postoperative Pain

The recent opioid crisis in America has generated broad interest in the development of opioid-sparing therapies in the perioperative setting. Temporary percutaneous, ultrasound-guided PNS is emerging as a potential opioid-sparing treatment of acute postoperative pain. While there have yet to be any large clinical trials examining the efficacy of treating acute postoperative pain, small feasibility studies have illustrated potential applications of this technique following various ambulatory orthopedic procedures: femoral nerve stimulation after anterior cruciate ligament reconstruction, subscapular nerve, and brachial plexus stimulation after rotator cuff repair, sciatic nerve stimulation after hallux valgus osteotomy and femoral and sciatic nerve stimulation after total knee arthroplasty.[51–55] A recent multicenter randomized control study comparing postoperative pain and opioid use in 32 patients receiving PNS and 34 patients receiving sham treatment found that the PNS group reported significantly less pain and opioid use in the week following surgery compared to the sham group.[56] One of the commercially available temporary PNS systems has FDA clearance for the treatment of both chronic and acute pain.[57]

Peripheral Nerve Stimulation Targeting of Motor Nerves

While sensory fibers are often the target of PNS, some clinicians have applied stimulation to the motor component of nerves to produce pain relief relief in the region of interest. For example, one study followed 9 patients with chronic axial low back pain who received a month of percutaneous stimulation localized to the medial branches of the dorsal rami causing contraction of the multifidus muscle.[58] One year after the cessation of treatment, most of the patients still reported reduced pain. A more recent study similarly examined the treatment of chronic axial low back pain with percutaneous stimulation of lumbar medial branch nerves; it found that most of the 51 patients who completed long-term follow-up visits experienced sustained decreases in pain and disability 1 year after finishing a 60-day stimulation period.[59]

Additionally, to treat hemiplegic shoulder pain in stroke survivors, clinicians have tried stimulating the axillary nerve.[60] Patients in one case series reported decreased pain 6, 12, and 24 months after beginning treatment with a fully implantable device. Shoulder pain stemming from various other causes including osteoarthritis and subacromial impingement syndrome (in addition to shoulder pain following rotator cuff repair, discussed elsewhere in this article) has also been responsive to the stimulation of motor nerves (the axillary and suprascapular nerves, specifically).[61]

Peripheral Nerve Stimulation for Neuroprosthetics

PNS is also under investigation as a means of creating neuroprosthetics: mechanical devices that can be controlled by or send sensory feedback to the patient's nervous system. In one study, researchers successfully used 16-contact nerve cuff electrodes to generate sensation that patients felt were originating from their missing limbs.[62] Another experiment demonstrated that PNS-induced and natural tactile stimuli are perceived comparably by patients.[63] In 2019, a team created a bionic hand that postamputation patients were able to control via 8 implanted electromyographic recording leads and that simulated sensory feedback by stimulating the median and ulnar nerves through Utah Slanted Electrode Arrays; the sensory feedback improved dexterity and functionality of the prosthetic device.[64]

Vagus Nerve Stimulation

Vagus nerve stimulation (VNS) has been explored as a therapeutic tool since the 19th century when it was discovered to have an anti-seizure effect.[65] Today, it is an FDA-approved option for the treatment of pharmacologically refractory epilepsy in patients who are not candidates for resective surgery. One commercially available device deploys stimulation to prevent seizures when it detects tachycardia predictive of imminent ictal activity.[66]

The FDA has also approved VNS for the treatment of depression, cluster headaches, and migraines, and a growing body of literature points to the potential benefits of this technique (both its invasive and transcutaneous implementations) in addressing other conditions. Some evolving areas of VNS research and proposed indications for the technique include:

- Ameliorating gait dysfunction and behavioral abnormalities in Parkinson's Disease.[67]
- Treating anxiety disorders.[68]
- Addressing motor and speech disorders in stroke survivors.[69]

- Promoting recovery following traumatic brain injury.[68]
- Countering cognitive disorders and memory issues in contexts such as Alzheimer's Disease.[68]
- Improving social functioning in patients with autism spectrum disorder.[68]
- Preventing systemic inflammatory response syndrome and postoperative ileus.[70]
- Managing inflammatory bowel disease.[71]
- Additional pain-related applications of PNS
- Stimulation of the occipital nerve to treat fibromyalgia.[72]

Additional Non–pain-related Applications of Peripheral Nerve Stimulation

- Percutaneous stimulation of the hypoglossal nerve and ansa cervicalis to treat obstructive sleep apnea.[73,74]
- Percutaneous stimulation of the tibial nerve to treat overactive bladder syndrome.[75]

SUMMARY

PNS is a powerful therapy for numerous pain conditions that are unresponsive to conventional forms of treatment. Procedural and technical innovations are rendering this technique progressively less invasive and disruptive, vastly expanding the list of possible indications. Advances in PNS are occurring rapidly, but in many cases, the efficacy of novel applications of neurostimulation has to be fully established with large randomized controlled trials. As such, it is important for clinicians treating patients suffering from intractable pain to be aware of recent directions in PNS research so they can remain abreast of emerging clinical evidence.

CLINICS CARE POINTS

- Patients with chronic, medically refractory neuropathic pain in a peripheral nerve distribution may be considered for PNS.
- Craniofacial PNS is typically performed using surface landmarks and/or fluoroscopy to assist in electrode placement.
- PNS elsewhere is typically performed using ultrasound guidance to assist in electrode placement and to avoid injury to adjacent structures.
- Most new PNS systems do not use IPGs, but use external generators instead.

- Motor PNS can be helpful for certain forms of low back pain, postsurgical shoulder pain, and poststroke pain.
- As for other forms of neuromodulation, PNS systems may use tonic as well as newer waveforms.
- PNS may also be used to treat several nonpain conditions, such as depression, obstructive sleep apnea, overactive bladder, mood disorders, and inflammatory bowel disease.

CONFLICT OF INTEREST DISCLOSURE

H.P. Fogel has no relevant commercial conflicts of interest to disclose. C.J. Winfree has no relevant commercial conflicts of interest to disclose.

REFERENCES

1. Shelden CH, Pudenz RH, Doyle J. Electrical control of facial pain. Am J Surg 1967;114(2):209–12.
2. Wall PD, Swert WH. Temporary abolition of pain in man. Science 1967;155(3758):108–9.
3. Melzack R, Wall PD. Pain mechanisms: a new theory. Science 1965;150(3699):971–9.
4. Lin T, Gargya A, Singh H, et al. Mechanism of peripheral nerve stimulation in chronic pain. Pain Med 2020;21(Suppl 1):S6.
5. Strand NH, D'Souza R, Wie C, et al. Mechanism of action of peripheral nerve stimulation. Curr Pain Headache Rep 2021;25(7):1–9.
6. Guo J, Jin H, Shi Z, et al. Sacral nerve stimulation improves colonic inflammation mediated by autonomic-inflammatory cytokine mechanism in rats. Neurogastroenterol Motil 2019;31(10):e13676.
7. García-Magro N, Negredo P, Martin YB, et al. Modulation of mechanosensory vibrissal responses in the trigeminocervical complex by stimulation of the greater occipital nerve in a rat model of trigeminal neuropathic pain. J Headache Pain 2020;21(1):1–17.
8. Sun KF, Feng WW, Liu YP, et al. Electrical peripheral nerve stimulation relieves bone cancer pain by inducing Arc protein expression in the spinal cord dorsal horn. J Pain Res 2018;11:599–609.
9. Deer TR, Mekhail N, Provenzano D, et al. The appropriate use of neurostimulation of the spinal cord and peripheral nervous system for the treatment of chronic pain and ischemic diseases: the Neuromodulation Appropriateness Consensus Committee. Neuromodulation 2014;17(6):515–50.
10. Winfree CJ. Peripheral nerve stimulation for facial pain using conventional devices: indications and results. Prog Neurol Surg 2020;35:60–7.
11. Texakalidis P, Tora MS, Anthony CL, et al. Peripheral trigeminal branch stimulation for refractory facial pain: a single-center experience. Clin Neurol Neurosurg 2020;194:105819.
12. Han R, Guo G, Ni Y, et al. Clinical efficacy of short-term peripheral nerve stimulation in management of facial pain associated with herpes zoster ophthalmicus. Front Neurosci 2020;14:574713.
13. Li C, White TG, Shah KA, et al. Percutaneous trigeminal nerve stimulation induces cerebral vasodilation in a dose-dependent manner. Neurosurgery 2021;88(6):E529–36.
14. Sweet JA, Mitchell LS, Narouze S, et al. Occipital nerve stimulation for the treatment of patients with medically refractory occipital neuralgia: congress of neurological surgeons systematic review and evidence-based guideline. Neurosurgery 2015;77(3):332–41.
15. Slavin Kv, Isagulyan ED, Gomez C, et al. Occipital nerve stimulation. Neurosurg Clin N Am 2019;30(2):211–7.
16. Raoul S, Nguyen JM, Kuhn E, et al. Efficacy of occipital nerve stimulation to treat refractory occipital headaches: a single-institution study of 60 patients. Neuromodulation 2020;23(6):789–95.
17. Joswig H, Abdallat M, Karapetyan V, et al. Long-term experience with occipital and supraorbital nerve stimulation for the various headache disorders-a retrospective institutional case series of 96 patients. World Neurosurg 2021;151:e472–83.
18. Kapural L, Yu C, Doust MW, et al. Comparison of 10-kHz high-frequency and traditional low-frequency spinal cord stimulation for the treatment of chronic back and leg pain: 24-month results from a multi-center, randomized, controlled pivotal trial. Neurosurgery 2016;79(5):667–76.
19. North JM, Hong KSJ, Cho PY. Clinical outcomes of 1 kHz subperception spinal cord stimulation in implanted patients with failed paresthesia-based stimulation: results of a prospective randomized controlled trial. Neuromodulation 2016;19(7):731–7.
20. Finch P, Drummond P. High-frequency peripheral nerve stimulation for craniofacial pain. Prog Neurol Surgery 2020;35:85–95.
21. Van Buyten JP, Smet I, Devos M, et al. High-frequency supraorbital nerve stimulation with a novel wireless minimally invasive device for posttraumatic neuralgia: a case report. Pain Pract 2019;19(4):435–9.
22. Finch P, Price L, Drummond P. High-frequency (10 kHz) electrical stimulation of peripheral nerves for treating chronic pain: a double-blind trial of presence vs absence of stimulation. Neuromodulation 2019;22(5):529–36.
23. Soin A, Syed Shah N, Fang ZP. High-frequency electrical nerve block for postamputation pain: a pilot study. Neuromodulation 2015;18(3):197–205.
24. Manning A, Ortega RG, Moir L, et al. Burst or conventional peripheral nerve field stimulation for

treatment of neuropathic facial pain. Neuromodulation 2019;22(5):645–52.

25. Garcia-Ortega R, Edwards T, Moir L, et al. Burst occipital nerve stimulation for chronic migraine and chronic cluster headache. Neuromodulation 2019;22(5):638–44.

26. Huntoon MA, Burgher AH. Ultrasound-guided permanent implantation of peripheral nerve stimulation (PNS) system for neuropathic pain of the extremities: original cases and outcomes. Pain Med 2009;10(8):1369–77.

27. Chan I, Brown AR, Park K, et al. Ultrasound-guided, percutaneous peripheral nerve stimulation: technical note. Neurosurgery 2010;67(3 Suppl Operative):ons136-9.

28. Regnier SM, Chen J, Gabriel RA, et al. A review of the StimRouter ® peripheral neuromodulation system for chronic pain management. Pain Manag 2021;11(3):227–36.

29. Mainkar O, Sollo CA, Chen G, et al. Pilot study in temporary peripheral nerve stimulation in oncologic pain. Neuromodulation 2020;23(6):819.

30. Salmasi V, Olatoye OO, Terkawi AS, et al. Peripheral nerve stimulation for occipital neuralgia. Pain Med 2020;21(Suppl 1):S13–7.

31. Mainkar O, Singh H, Gargya A, et al. Ultrasound-guided peripheral nerve stimulation of cervical, thoracic, and lumbar spinal nerves for dermatomal pain: a case series. Neuromodulation 2021;24(6):1059–66.

32. Gilmore C, Ilfeld B, Rosenow J, et al. Percutaneous peripheral nerve stimulation for the treatment of chronic neuropathic postamputation pain: a multicenter, randomized, placebo-controlled trial. Reg Anesth Pain Med 2019;44(6):637–45.

33. Ilfeld BM, Grant SA, Gilmore CA, et al. Neurostimulation for postsurgical analgesia: a novel system enabling ultrasound-guided percutaneous peripheral nerve stimulation. Pain Pract 2017;17(7):892.

34. Stokey BG, Weiner RL, Slavin KV, et al. Peripheral nerve stimulation for facial pain using wireless devices. Prog Neurol Surg 2020;35:75–84.

35. Abd-Elsayed A. Wireless peripheral nerve stimulation for treatment of peripheral neuralgias. Neuromodulation 2020;23(6):827–30.

36. Billet B, Wynendaele R, Vanquathem NE. A novel minimally invasive wireless technology for neuromodulation via percutaneous intercostal nerve stimulation for post-herpetic neuralgia: a case report with short-term follow-up. Pain Pract 2018;18(3):374–9. https://doi.org/10.1111/PAPR.12607.

37. Herschkowitz D, Kubias J. Wireless peripheral nerve stimulation for complex regional pain syndrome type I of the upper extremity: a case illustration introducing a novel technology. Scand J Pain 2018;18(3):555–60.

38. Piech DK, Johnson BC, Shen K, et al. A wireless millimetre-scale implantable neural stimulator with ultrasonically powered bidirectional communication. Nat Biomed Eng 2020;4(2):207–22.

39. Deer TR, Eldabe S, Falowski SM, et al. Peripherally induced reconditioning of the central nervous system: a proposed mechanistic theory for sustained relief of chronic pain with percutaneous peripheral nerve stimulation. J Pain Res 2021;14:721.

40. Ilfeld BM, Gabriel RA, Saulino MF, et al. Infection rates of electrical leads used for percutaneous neurostimulation of the peripheral nervous system. Pain Pract 2017;17(6):753.

41. Shellock FG, Zare A, Ilfeld BM, et al. In vitro magnetic resonance imaging evaluation of fragmented, open-coil, percutaneous peripheral nerve stimulation leads. Neuromodulation 2018;21(3):276–83.

42. Sperry BP, Cheney CW, Kuo KT, et al. Percutaneous treatments for residual and/or phantom limb pain in adults with lower-extremity amputations: a narrative review. PM R 2021. https://doi.org/10.1002/PMRJ.12722.

43. Rauck RL, Kapural L, Cohen SP, et al. Peripheral nerve stimulation for the treatment of postamputation pain–a case report. Pain Pract 2012;12(8):649–55.

44. Rauck RL, Cohen SP, Gilmore CA, et al. Treatment of post-amputation pain with peripheral nerve stimulation. Neuromodulation 2014;17(2):188–97.

45. Meier K, Bendtsen TF, Sørensen JC, et al. Peripheral neuromodulation for the treatment of postamputation neuroma pain: a case report. A A Case Rep 2017;8(2):29–30.

46. Sondekoppam RV, Ip V, Tsui BCH. Feasibility of combining nerve stimulation and local anesthetic infusion to treat acute postamputation pain: a case report of a hybrid technique. A&A Pract 2021;15(6):e01487.

47. Agrawal NA, Gfrerer L, Heng M, et al. The use of peripheral nerve stimulation in conjunction with TMR for neuropathic pain. Plast Reconstr Surg Glob Open 2021;9(6):e3655.

48. Gilmore CA, Ilfeld BM, Rosenow JM, et al. Percutaneous 60-day peripheral nerve stimulation implant provides sustained relief of chronic pain following amputation: 12-month follow-up of a randomized, double-blind, placebo-controlled trial. Reg Anesth Pain Med 2019;45(1):44–51.

49. Jung MJ, Pritzlaff SG. Peripheral nerve stimulation for treatment of severe refractory upper extremity post-amputation pain. Neuromodulation 2021;24(6):1127–8.

50. Finneran JJ, Furnish T, Curran BP, et al. Percutaneous peripheral nerve stimulation of the brachial plexus for intractable phantom pain of the upper extremity: a case report. A&A Pract 2020;14(14):e01353.

51. Ilfeld BM, Said ET, Finneran JJ, et al. Ultrasound-guided percutaneous peripheral nerve stimulation: neuromodulation of the femoral nerve for postoperative analgesia following ambulatory anterior cruciate ligament reconstruction: a proof of concept study. Neuromodulation 2019;22(5):621–9.

52. Ilfeld BM, Finneran JJ, Gabriel RA, et al. Ultrasound-guided percutaneous peripheral nerve stimulation: Neuromodulation of the suprascapular nerve and brachial plexus for postoperative analgesia following ambulatory rotator cuff repair. A proof-of-concept study. Reg Anesth Pain Med 2019;44(3):310–8.

53. Ilfeld BM, Gabriel RA, Said ET, et al. Ultrasound-guided percutaneous peripheral nerve stimulation: neuromodulation of the sciatic nerve for postoperative analgesia following ambulatory foot surgery, a proof-of-concept study. Reg Anesth Pain Med 2018;43(6):580–9.

54. Ilfeld BM, Gilmore CA, Grant SA, et al. Ultrasound-guided percutaneous peripheral nerve stimulation for analgesia following total knee arthroplasty: a prospective feasibility study. J Orthopaedic Surg Res 2017;12(1):4.

55. Ilfeld BM, Ball ST, Gabriel RA, et al. A feasibility study of percutaneous peripheral nerve stimulation for the treatment of postoperative pain following total knee arthroplasty. Neuromodulation 2019;22(5):653–60.

56. Ilfeld BM, Plunkett A, Vijjeswarapu AM, et al. Percutaneous peripheral nerve stimulation (Neuromodulation) for postoperative pain: a randomized, sham-controlled pilot study. Anesthesiology 2021;135(1):95–110.

57. Gabriel RA, Ilfeld BM. Acute postoperative pain management with percutaneous peripheral nerve stimulation: the SPRINT neuromodulation system. Expert Rev Med Devices 2021;18(2):145–50.

58. Gilmore CA, Kapural L, McGee MJ, et al. Percutaneous peripheral nerve stimulation for chronic low back pain: prospective case series with 1 year of sustained relief following short-term implant. Pain Pract 2020;20(3):310.

59. Gilmore CA, Desai MJ, Hopkins TJ, et al. Treatment of chronic axial back pain with 60-day percutaneous medial branch PNS: Primary end point results from a prospective, multicenter study. Pain Pract 2021;21(8):877–89.

60. Wilson RD, Bennett ME, Nguyen VQC, et al. Fully implantable peripheral nerve stimulation for hemiplegic shoulder pain: a multi-site case series with two-year follow-up. Neuromodulation 2018;21(3):290–5.

61. Mazzola A, Spinner D. Ultrasound-guided peripheral nerve stimulation for shoulder pain: anatomic review and assessment of the current clinical evidence. Available at: www.painphysicianjournal.com. Accessed November 30, 2021.

62. Christie BP, Graczyk EL, Charkhkar H, et al. High-density peripheral nerve cuffs restore natural sensation to individuals with lower-limb amputations. J Neural Eng 2018;15(5):056002.

63. Christie BP, Graczyk EL, Charkhkar H, et al. Visuo-tactile synchrony of stimulation-induced sensation and natural somatosensation. J Neural Eng 2019;16(3):036025.

64. George JA, Kluger DT, Davis TS, et al. Biomimetic sensory feedback through peripheral nerve stimulation improves dexterous use of a bionic hand. Sci Robotics 2019;4(32):eaax2352.

65. Broncel A, Bocian R, Kłos-Wojtczak P, et al. Vagal nerve stimulation as a promising tool in the improvement of cognitive disorders. Brain Res Bull 2020;155:37–47.

66. Hamilton P, Soryal I, Dhahri P, et al. Clinical outcomes of VNS therapy with AspireSR ® (including cardiac-based seizure detection) at a large complex epilepsy and surgery centre. Seizure 2018;58:120–6.

67. Sigurdsson HP, Raw R, Hunter H, et al. Noninvasive vagus nerve stimulation in Parkinson's disease: current status and future prospects. Expert Rev Med Devices 2021;18(10):971–84.

68. Wang Y, Zhan G, Cai Z, et al. Vagus nerve stimulation in brain diseases: therapeutic applications and biological mechanisms. Neurosci Biobehav Rev 2021;127:37–53.

69. Morrison RA, Hays SA, Kilgard MP. Vagus nerve stimulation as a potential adjuvant to rehabilitation for post-stroke motor speech disorders. Front Neurosci 2021;15:715928.

70. van Beekum CJ, Willis MA, von Websky MW, et al. Electrical vagus nerve stimulation as a prophylaxis for SIRS and postoperative ileus. Auton Neurosci 2021;235:102857.

71. Cheng J, Shen H, Chowdhury R, et al. Potential of electrical neuromodulation for inflammatory bowel disease. Inflamm Bowel Dis 2020;26(8):1119–30.

72. Plazier M, Dekelver I, Vanneste S, et al. Occipital nerve stimulation in fibromyalgia: a double-blind placebo-controlled pilot study with a six-month follow-up. Neuromodulation 2014;17(3):256–64.

73. Olson MD, Junna MR. Hypoglossal nerve stimulation therapy for the treatment of obstructive sleep apnea. Neurotherapeutics 2021;18(1):91–9.

74. Kent DT, Zealear D, Schwartz AR. Ansa cervicalis stimulation: a new direction in neurostimulation for OSA. Chest 2021;159(3):1212–21.

75. Wang M, Jian Z, Ma Y, et al. Percutaneous tibial nerve stimulation for overactive bladder syndrome: a systematic review and meta-analysis. Int Urogynecol J 2020;31(12):2457–71.

Focused Ultrasound for Chronic Pain

Jonathan Bao, BS[a], Thomas Tangney, BS[a], Julie G. Pilitsis, MD, PhD[a,b,*]

KEYWORDS

- Focused ultrasound • Pain • Ablation • Neuromodulation

KEY POINTS

- Focused ultrasound can be used for ablation, neuromodulation, and opening of the blood-brain barrier to treat various disorders, including chronic pain.
- Limited clinical applications have been approved and have been mostly centered on ablative focused ultrasound for chronic neuropathic pain.
- Additional clinical studies are needed to expand usage for chronic pain and revolutionize neurosurgical treatments.

INTRODUCTION

Chronic pain affects approximately 20.4% of adults in the United States and puts a significant economic burden on the US economy.[1] At present, many treatments do not work for all patients, require invasive surgery, or result in the use of opioids. One promising treatment technique has emerged in recent years using focused ultrasound (FUS) technology. FUS has grown in its clinical applications in the past 70 years and has shown potential in the treatment of many neurologic disorders including neuropathic pain.[2–4] FUS uses various focusing techniques to concentrate and converge ultrasound waves on a small region; this allows for the energy to be targeted to specific areas such as brain structures or the dorsal root ganglia (DRG) without damaging or altering other regions. In addition, advancements in FUS technology have enabled its use noninvasively, making it an attractive treatment modality for many neurologic disorders.[5–8]

Current utilizations of FUS are categorized into 3 based on the FUS parameters: (1) tissue ablation, (2) neuromodulation, and (3) alterations of blood-brain barrier (BBB) permeability. Most clinical work in recent years has revolved around the development of FUS technology for noninvasive tissue ablation. However, further research is needed to effectively use FUS clinically to treat patients. Here we discuss clinical applications and advancements of FUS technology in the treatment of chronic pain. In addition, this review delineates limitations within the field and future studies needed to overcome these barriers and expand the usage of FUS into neurosurgical clinics.

FOCUSED ULTRASOUND

Ultrasound is a mechanical wave that has a frequency greater than 20 kHz (the limit for sound detection by the human ear) and possesses the ability to transmit mechanical energy. These ultrasound waves, like other mechanical waves, are subject to alterations when traveling through different media. Within biological tissues, alterations are observed at different degrees in varying tissues and are particularly noticed when traveling through structures like the skull or at bone-tissue interfaces where ultrasound can be significantly attenuated.[9] To produce ultrasound waves, devices generally use a generator to create an electrical signal, an amplifier to magnify the signal,

[a] Department of Neuroscience and Experimental Therapeutics, Albany Medical College, 43 New Scotland Ave, Albany, NY 12208, USA; [b] Department of Neurosurgery, Albany Medical Center, 43 New Scotland Ave, Albany, NY 12208, USA
* Corresponding author. AMC Neurosurgery Group, 47 New Scotland Avenue, MC 10 Physicians Pavilion, 1st Floor, Albany, NY 12208.
E-mail address: jpilitsis@yahoo.com

Neurosurg Clin N Am 33 (2022) 331–338
https://doi.org/10.1016/j.nec.2022.02.010
1042-3680/22/© 2022 Elsevier Inc. All rights reserved.

and a transducer to transform the electrical signal into a mechanical sound wave.

Traditional uses for ultrasound have generally revolved around its visualization abilities. However, with the development of the first FUS device by the Fry brothers, the clinical applications of ultrasound have greatly expanded (**Table 1**). The Fry brothers are credited with some of the most influential work in FUS during the 1950s and the 1960s because they performed numerous studies in mammalian models.[10–12] In particular, they studied the ablative abilities of FUS, including a partial ablation of the basal ganglia.[11] However, these studies required burr holes or craniotomies to effectively transmit the ultrasound waves deep into brain tissue. Challenges in delivering FUS through the skull remained until the 1990s when advancements in magnetic resonance thermometry, transducer design, and phase corrections enabled the ability for FUS to be delivered noninvasively.[5–8]

The first documented biological effects of ultrasound were observed by Langevin when he found that high-intensity ultrasound was able to debilitate fish that swam through its beams.[13] Following this discovery, extensive study has been performed to fully understand the mechanism through which FUS can exhibit biological effects on the nervous system and other tissues. FUS is not completely understood and is believed to exert its effects through 2 mechanisms: (1) thermal changes and (2) mechanical distortions produced by the ultrasound waves. Both effects depend on the dose of FUS applied to these regions, inherent tissue properties, and the duration of ultrasound treatment. Ablative FUS can increase tissue temperatures to greater than of 55°C, which can cause cellular damage and protein denaturation.[13–16] In contrast, lower-intensity FUS produces mechanical disturbances through alterations of membrane proteins, cavitations, mechanical pressure, and also disruptions of barriers, such as the BBB, without significant temperature changes.[13,17–22] Although mechanical and thermal changes are considered separately, application of FUS often causes both changes to occur simultaneously and makes it difficult to isolate the effects.

ABLATIVE FOCUSED ULTRASOUND

Ablative FUS was first clinically studied in brain tumors.[23,24] Following this success, usages of FUS in this field have expanded to treat Parkinson disease, essential tremor, and neuropathic pain.[2,3,25,26] This application of FUS is performed noninvasively through a transcranial magnetic resonance-guided (MR-guided) mechanism. At present, the US Food and Drug Administration has approved the usage of ExAblate system (Insightec, Tirat Carmel, Israel) for transcranial MR-guided FUS in humans.

Table 1
Relevant studies in pain

Study	Type of Study	Type of FUS	Findings/Relevance
Martin et al,[2] 2009	Clinical	Ablative	Central thalamic lesion study to demonstrate precise targeting and no short-term adverse events or complications
Jeanmonod et al,[3] 2012	Clinical	Ablative	Lesions of central thalamic nucleus led to immediate pain relief in some patients suffering from chronic neuropathic pain
Hameroff et al,[45] 2013	Clinical	Neuromodulatory	FUS at frontal cortex showed in affective ratings pain and nonsignificant changes in NRS
Badran et al,[46] 2020	Clinical	Neuromodulatory	MR-guided FUS targeted to right anterior thalamus demonstrated diminished thermal sensitivity
Mainprize et al,[66] 2019	Clinical	BBB drug delivery	BBB disruption can be used to deliver drugs such as chemotherapeutic agents
Airan et al,[69] 2017	Basic science	BBB drug delivery	Delivery of drugs through nanoparticles that break down in response to FUS and do not require BBB disruption

Abbreviation: NRS, numeric rating scale.

For treatment of chronic pain, 2 clinical studies have been performed. In the first study, 9 patients with chronic refractory neuropathic pain received central thalamotomies using FUS.[2] An accurate thermal ablation of approximately 4 mm was created. Tissue temperatures reached between 51°C and 60°C following delivery of 10 to 20 seconds of continuous treatment. These lesions were visualized with MRI immediately after and 48 hours following the procedure with no side effects or adverse events reported at the time. This work demonstrated feasibility and safety. Following this study, this same group expanded their clinical study to another 11 patients.[3] In this follow-up study, lesions of 3 to 4 mm in diameter were created in the central lateral thalamic nucleus and therapy administered using real-time MR thermometry. Six patients experienced immediate pain relief following the ablation that persisted in future follow-up appointments. However, one patient was reported to have suffered from right-sided dysmetria in the arms and legs and dysarthria due to a thalamic bleed at the ablation site. These neurologic deficits had improved at 1-year follow-up.

Overall, patients demonstrated a 49% improvement in pain on the visual analog scale (VAS) at a 3-month follow-up and 57% improvement at a 12-month follow-up. In addition, some patients reported moderate reductions in pain medication usage. Furthermore, electroencephalography (EEG) studies indicated that patients had reduced spectral power in all frequency ranges at 3 and 12 month after ablation and approached values similar to healthy volunteers. Studies like these demonstrate the tremendous promise FUS has in ablative applications for pain treatment.

However, ablative FUS use has been limited at this time to central brain structures. This limitation is due to the high surface brain temperatures that may occur when targeting more superficial and lateral brain structures.[27–29] This effect occurs with increased reflection and decreased penetrance of ultrasound waves associated with superficial structures that can lead to increased heating of the brain surface.[30] These effects may in part be due to FUS parameters, which may be improved in the future. In addition, FUS ablation procedures are not able to efficiently ablate large areas due to potential adverse effects in the surrounding brain regions.[31,32] Furthermore, patients may be unable to tolerate the duration of treatment of these cases.

With improved technological capabilities and further research to optimize treatment parameters, ablative FUS can be used to target additional brain regions and replace current treatment technologies used in the neurosurgical field. With the ability to target additional structures, other brain regions important for pain processing such as the cingulate cortex can be used to achieve pain relief. In addition, FUS may offer benefit over stereotactic radiosurgery due to its lack of radiation.[33,34]

NEUROMODULATION WITH FOCUSED ULTRASOUND

Neuromodulation therapy is used to alter neuronal activity most commonly through electrical stimulation and can treat a variety of disorders including chronic pain. FUS applied with lower intensities and pulsing holds promise for a nonelectrical means of modulating both the peripheral nervous system (PNS) and central nervous system (CNS).[35] FUS-induced reversible and temporary modifications of neuronal activity have been observed early on during studies of FUS but gained traction only recently.[36–38] Current work has used in vivo and in vitro preclinical models. Although its effects are not fully understood, FUS is believed to exert its neuromodulatory effects through a combination of mechanosensitive ion channel activation and mechanical disturbances of the plasma membrane.[20,39] There have been a limited number of human clinical trials looking at the effects of modulatory FUS in epilepsy, Alzheimer disease, anxiety, and brain injury.[30]

Modulation of the CNS with FUS in humans began in studies examining changes in sensory perception. Two studies examined the effects of FUS applied on the somatosensory cortex and observed that stimulation led to numbness/tingling and could suppress evoked action potentials in the median nerve.[40,41] Both the FUS-induced sensations and neuronal inhibition were confirmed in another study by Legon and colleagues who demonstrated that primary motor cortex stimulation also produced similar changes.[42] For pain, 2 clinical studies have been performed. The first study examined 31 patients with chronic pain who were treated with transcranial ultrasound targeted at the posterior frontal cortex and demonstrated that patients had significant improvements in subjective affect and slight improvements in their numeric rating scale score.[43] However, this was a proof-of-concept study and did not eliminate the potential for confounding factors because it was a crossover trial. This study also did not verify brain targeting and/or examine alterations in brain activity following the treatment. The second study used MR-guided pulsed transcranial FUS on the right anterior thalamus in 19 healthy subjects and found that treatment

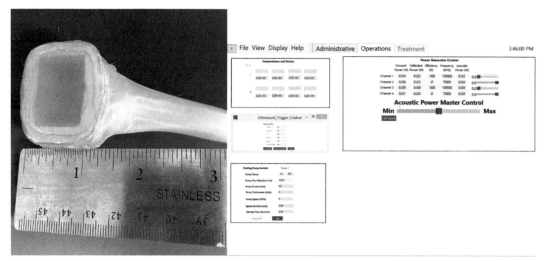

Fig. 1. FUS probe and FUS software (Acoustic MedSystems, Savoy, IL, USA) used for rodent studies of FUS neuromodulation.

significantly diminished thermal pain sensitivity.[44] Similar to the first study, this was also a proof-of-concept study and thus lacked the sample size and proper study design to make significant conclusions. However, taken together both demonstrate premise for future work.

Work with FUS in the periphery has largely been performed in animal studies. Various groups have demonstrated that FUS stimulation produces an intensity- and time-dependent effect that can alter neuronal activity and induce tactile sensations.[45–47] Our group has investigated the effects of external low-intensity pulsed FUS (liFUS) in reversing pain behavior in multiple animal models of neuropathic pain both with internal and external liFUS. We have demonstrated the ability of liFUS to improve sensory thresholds and pain behavior for up to 3 to 5 days following treatment in rodents without producing tachyphylaxis or histologic damage to tissue.[48–50] We have shown that conduction latency of the common peroneal nerve decreases with treatment to the L5 DRG.[51] We have demonstrated similar results in swine where we have effectively developed a chronic neuropathic pain model.[52,53] Animals had improved mechanical and thermal thresholds and normalization in nerve conduction velocities following treatment with liFUS without any histologic damage.[52] We are now investigating changes in neuronal activity in supraspinal pain processing regions. This work is important in eventually translating this treatment method into the clinic for usage. As a treatment modality, this device can be easily administered to patients in a clinic setting without the need for an operating room or MRI equipment, significantly reducing cost and time for treatments (**Fig. 1**).

In addition, this treatment can be delivered non-invasively, can overcome the addictive nature of opioids, and can be repeatedly used without the development of tolerance. Although our current studies have mostly targeted DRG and the occipital nerve, FUS can be targeted to other peripheral nerve structures to provide more specific pain relief. These capabilities can then potentially replace pulsed radiofrequency (RF), which has been investigated as a peripheral nerve treatment modality.[54,55–59] RF has been demonstrated to provide short-term pain relief, but it is a procedure that remains largely invasive and can have potentially serious side effects due to thermal damage to surrounding tissues.[60,55–61] Thus, FUS can overcome these weaknesses and has great potential in neuromodulation for chronic pain.

BLOOD-BRAIN MODIFICATION/DRUG DELIVERY USING FOCUSED ULTRASOUND

The BBB is a highly selective interface that limits permeability of certain potentially toxic or large hydrophilic molecules between the circulatory system and CNS. FUS waves have been shown to disrupt tight junctions in endothelial cells in the BBB increasing the permeability to agents that were previously nonpenetrable.[32] FUS is capable of altering the permeability of BBB for up to 24 hours before returning it to previous state.[62,63] This technique has also shown the capability of increasing drug concentration in a specific targeted area of brain tissue.[62,64] This method of increasing delivery of drugs has the potential to lower dosages of pain medication needed, reducing side effects and chances of toxicity.

FUS can also be applied noninvasively through the skull and does not require surgical intervention, eliminating the risk from those procedures. Treatment using this technique could also spare nontargeted brain tissue or other organs from high drug concentrations. Furthermore, the capability of FUS to open the blood-spinal cord barrier has been demonstrated suggesting the possibility of targeting pain along any part of the CNS[65]; this could also have a benefit in reducing side effects because targeted delivery could lower the systemic dose while still maintaining an effect at the targeted site. A study on patients with tumor using MR-guided FUS demonstrated safe opening of the BBB and administration of chemotherapy.[66] It has been shown in rat models that albumin permeability in BBB increases after transcranial pulsed FUS and that the duration of effect can be adjusted due to interval between repeat sonications.[67,68] This observation suggests that the extent of drug delivery can be controlled through the timing of treatment.

Another potential strategy for increasing delivery of agents across the BBB with FUS is ultrasound-mediated drug uncaging from nanoparticle carriers. There is evidence that this technique, using developed biodegradable nanoparticles, allows for particles that cross the BBB passively and labeled inert by nanoparticles to become active through ultrasound without hemorrhage or BBB disruption[69]; this potentially allows the benefit of increasing delivery of pain medication without sacrificing the functions of the BBB due to disruption during the use of ultrasound, resulting in focal control for delivery through noninvasive means. Although this technique requires lipophilic agents, there are many pain medications that fall under this requirement such as gabapentin.

Medications such as gabapentin have been shown to have a moderate benefit on neuropathic pain but have also shown significant adverse side effects.[70] Modulation of the BBB could allow greater concentrations to reach the CNS. Possible reduction of dosage with FUS may then limit adverse side effects such as somnolence, dizziness, and/or ataxia along. Furthermore, the increased concentration may reduce the duration between treatment initiation and effect. Similarly in the end-of-life patient who requires high-dose opioids for pain relief, BBB alterations may allow opioids to be used at doses that are effective but do not lead to somnolence or respiratory depression. This technique also has the potential to target locally reducing the possibility of interactions with other drugs.[71]

Despite the promise some studies have shown for using FUS to alter BBB permeability to increase drug delivery, there are current limitations to this treatment. New safety profiles will need to be established to reduce risks of drug toxicity in the brain.[72] With the use of preformed microbubble ultrasound contrast agent in conjunction with FUS, there is evidence that this technique can be used safely.[73–75] However, it has been shown that FUS opening of BBB with this contrast agent induces local inflammatory response.[76] Further studies regarding FUS, BBB permeability, and drug delivery will be needed to refine the parameters for this technique and determine safety and efficacy. The application of these techniques for chronic pain treatment is also not well studied and will require more investigation.

SUMMARY AND FUTURE DIRECTIONS

FUS has tremendous clinical promise and has seen great progress in its use for ablative, neuromodulatory, and BBB disruption for drug delivery as treatments for various neurologic disorders. Although each has been used successfully in human trials, the greatest challenge remains to unlock and expand its full potential to treat a wider variety of diseases including chronic pain; this includes the need for technological advancement to target more brain structures and more efficiently open the BBB, mechanistic studies to fully use neuromodulation of the CNS or PNS, and optimization studies to fully develop ultrasound parameters to maximize its effects. Despite these challenges, current studies of FUS have demonstrated the ability to treat chronic pain or chronic pain behavior and show potential for expanded use in this field. In addition, FUS, unlike other treatment modalities for chronic pain, combines the ability to provide noninvasive treatment, targets deep structures, accurately localizes targets, and avoids problems with addiction and other side effects commonly associated with pain medications. Thus, this provides an unparalleled flexibility that makes it an ideal and attractive treatment option for chronic pain that can revolutionize the neurosurgical clinic.

CLINICS CARE POINTS

- Ablative FUS can destroy brain tissue in order to treat chronic pain; however, this tissue destruction is mostly limited to central brain structures due to increased brain surface temperatures found when targeting more superficial and lateral areas.

- CNS neuromodulation has been clinically studied in 2 proof-of-concept studies which found that FUS improved pain scores, subjective affect, and thermal pain sensitivity.

- PNS neuromodulation has been studied in multiple animal models of chronic pain and has demonstrated improved sensory thresholds and pain behavior. Additional work has examined the mechanism of action and future studies look to translate these findings into human usage.

- Disruption of the blood-brain barrier and targeted drug delivery utilizing FUS provides increased flexibility and versatility in accurately delivering appropriate drug doses to many regions including areas such as the brain which were previously difficult to target.

CONFLICTS OF INTEREST

Dr J.G. Pilitsis is a consultant for Boston Scientific, Nevro, Medtronic, Saluda, and Abbott and receives grant support from Medtronic, Boston Scientific, Abbott, Nevro, NIH 2R01CA166379-06, and NIH U44NS115111. She is the medical advisor for Aim Medical Robotics and Karuna and has stock equity. All other authors have no further or distinct disclosures.

REFERENCES

1. Dahlhamer J, Lucas J, Zelaya C, et al. Prevalence of Chronic Pain and High-Impact Chronic Pain Among Adults - United States, 2016. MMWR Morb Mortal Wkly Rep 2018;67(36):1001–6.

2. Martin E, Jeanmonod D, Morel A, et al. High-intensity focused ultrasound for noninvasive functional neurosurgery. Ann Neurol 2009;66(6):858–61.

3. Jeanmonod D, Werner B, Morel A, et al. Transcranial magnetic resonance imaging-guided focused ultrasound: noninvasive central lateral thalamotomy for chronic neuropathic pain. Neurosurg Focus 2012; 32(1):E1.

4. Meyers R, Fry FJ, Fry WJ, et al. Determination of topologic human brain representations and modifications of signs and symptoms of some neurologic disorders by the use of high level ultrasound. Neurology 1960;10(3):271–7.

5. Hynynen K, McDannold N, Clement G, et al. Preclinical testing of a phased array ultrasound system for MRI-guided noninvasive surgery of the brain–a primate study. Eur J Radiol 2006;59(2): 149–56.

6. Hynynen K, Sun J. Trans-skull ultrasound therapy: the feasibility of using image-derived skull thickness information to correct the phase distortion. IEEE Trans Ultrason Ferroelectr Freq Control 1999;46(3): 752–5.

7. Pernot M, Aubry JF, Tanter M, et al. In vivo transcranial brain surgery with an ultrasonic time reversal mirror. J Neurosurg 2007;106(6):1061–6.

8. Cline HE, Schenck JF, Hynynen K, et al. MR-guided focused ultrasound surgery. J Comput Assist Tomogr 1992;16(6):956–65.

9. Pinton G, Aubry JF, Bossy E, et al. Attenuation, scattering, and absorption of ultrasound in the skull bone. Med Phys 2012;39(1):299–307.

10. Fry FJ. Precision high intensity focusing ultrasonic machines for surgery. Am J Phys Med 1958;37(3): 152–6.

11. Fry WJ, Barnard JW, Fry EJ, et al. Ultrasonic lesions in the mammalian central nervous system. Science 1955;122(3168):517–8.

12. Fry WJ, Meyers R. Ultrasonic method of modifying brain st ructures. Confin Neurol 1962;22:315–27.

13. O'Brien WD Jr. Ultrasound-biophysics mechanisms. Prog Biophys Mol Biol 2007;93(1–3):212–55.

14. Krishna V, Sammartino F, Rezai A. A Review of the Current Therapies, Challenges, and Future Directions of Transcranial Focused Ultrasound Technology: Advances in Diagnosis and Treatment. JAMA Neurol 2018;75(2):246–54.

15. Rossmanna C, Haemmerich D. Review of temperature dependence of thermal properties, dielectric properties, and perfusion of biological tissues at hyperthermic and ablation temperatures. Crit Rev Biomed Eng 2014;42(6):467–92.

16. Seip R, Ebbini ES. Noninvasive estimation of tissue temperature response to heating fields using diagnostic ultrasound. IEEE Trans Biomed Eng 1995; 42(8):828–39.

17. Dalecki D. Mechanical bioeffects of ultrasound. Annu Rev Biomed Eng 2004;6:229–48.

18. Izadifar Z, Babyn P, Chapman D. Mechanical and Biological Effects of Ultrasound: A Review of Present Knowledge. Ultrasound Med Biol 2017;43(6): 1085–104.

19. Bakay L, Ballantine HT Jr, Hueter TF, et al. Ultrasonically produced changes in the blood-brain barrier. AMA Arch Neurol Psychiatry 1956;76(5):457–67.

20. Kubanek J, Shukla P, Das A, et al. Ultrasound Elicits Behavioral Responses through Mechanical Effects on Neurons and Ion Channels in a Simple Nervous System. J Neurosci 2018;38(12):3081–91.

21. Patrick JT, Nolting MN, Goss SA, et al. Ultrasound and the blood-brain barrier. Adv Exp Med Biol 1990;267:369–81.

22. Sirsi S, Borden M. Microbubble Compositions, Properties and Biomedical Applications. Bubble Sci Eng Technol 2009;1(1–2):3–17.

23. McDannold N, Clement GT, Black P, et al. Transcranial magnetic resonance imaging- guided focused

ultrasound surgery of brain tumors: initial findings in 3 patients. Neurosurgery 2010;66(2):323–32.

24. Ram Z, Cohen ZR, Harnof S, et al. Magnetic resonance imaging-guided, high-intensity focused ultrasound for brain tumor therapy. Neurosurgery 2006; 59(5):949–55.

25. Na YC, Chang WS, Jung HH, et al. Unilateral magnetic resonance-guided focused ultrasound pallidotomy for Parkinson disease. Neurology 2015; 85(6):549–51.

26. Elias WJ, Huss D, Voss T, et al. A pilot study of focused ultrasound thalamotomy for essential tremor. N Engl J Med 2013;369(7):640–8.

27. Top CB, White PJ, McDannold NJ. Nonthermal ablation of deep brain targets: A simulation study on a large animal model. Med Phys 2016;43(2):870–82.

28. Aubry JF, Tanter M. MR-Guided Transcranial Focused Ultrasound. Adv Exp Med Biol 2016;880:97–111.

29. Odeen H, de Bever J, Almquist S, et al. Treatment envelope evaluation in transcranial magnetic resonance-guided focused ultrasound utilizing 3D MR thermometry. J Ther Ultrasound 2014;2:19.

30. McDannold N, Zhang YZ, Power C, et al. Nonthermal ablation with microbubble-enhanced focused ultrasound close to the optic tract without affecting nerve function. J Neurosurg 2013;119(5):1208–20.

31. Leinenga G, Langton C, Nisbet R, et al. Ultrasound treatment of neurological diseases–current and emerging applications. Nat Rev Neurol 2016;12(3): 161–74.

32. Todd N, McDannold N, Borsook D. Targeted manipulation of pain neural networks: The potential of focused ultrasound for treatment of chronic pain. Neurosci Biobehav Rev 2020;115:238–50.

33. Roberts DG, Pouratian N. Stereotactic Radiosurgery for the Treatment of Chronic Intractable Pain: A Systematic Review. Oper Neurosurg (Hagerstown) 2017;13(5):543–51.

34. Singh R, Davis J, Sharma S. Stereotactic Radiosurgery for Trigeminal Neuralgia: A Retrospective Multi-Institutional Examination of Treatment Outcomes. Cureus 2016;8(4):e554.

35. Fetcko K, Lukas RV, Watson GA, et al. Survival and complications of stereotactic radiosurgery: A systematic review of stereotactic radiosurgery for newly diagnosed and recurrent high-grade gliomas. Medicine (Baltimore) 2017;96(43):e8293.

36. Khraiche ML, Phillips WB, Jackson N, et al. Ultrasound induced increase in excitability of single neurons. Annu Int Conf IEEE Eng Med Biol Soc 2008; 2008:4246–9.

37. Tufail Y, Matyushov A, Baldwin N, et al. Transcranial pulsed ultrasound stimulates intact brain circuits. Neuron 2010;66(5):681–94.

38. Harvey EN. The effect of high frequency sound waves on heart muscle and other irritable tissues. Am J Phys 1929;91(1):7.

39. Ballantine HT Jr, Bell E, Manlapaz J. Progress and problems in the neurological applications of focused ultrasound. J Neurosurg 1960;17:858–76.

40. Fry FJ, Ades HW, Fry WJ. Production of reversible changes in the central nervous system by ultrasound. Science 1958;127(3289):83–4.

41. Blackmore J, Shrivastava S, Sallet J, et al. Ultrasound Neuromodulation: A Review of Results, Mechanisms and Safety. Ultrasound Med Biol 2019;45(7): 1509–36.

42. Lee W, Kim H, Jung Y, et al. Image-guided transcranial focused ultrasound stimulates human primary somatosensory cortex. Sci Rep 2015;5:8743.

43. Legon W, Sato TF, Opitz A, et al. Transcranial focused ultrasound modulates the activity of primary somatosensory cortex in humans. Nat Neurosci 2014;17(2):322–9.

44. Legon W, Bansal P, Tyshynsky R, et al. Transcranial focused ultrasound neuromodulation of the human primary motor cortex. Sci Rep 2018;8(1):10007.

45. Hameroff S, Trakas M, Duffield C, et al. Transcranial ultrasound (TUS) effects on mental states: a pilot study. Brain Stimul 2013;6(3):409–15.

46. Badran BW, Caulfield KA, Stomberg-Firestein S, et al. Sonication of the anterior thalamus with MRI-Guided transcranial focused ultrasound (tFUS) alters pain thresholds in healthy adults: A double-blind, sham-controlled study. Brain Stimul 2020;13(6):1805–12.

47. Chye CL, Liang CL, Lu K, et al. Pulsed radiofrequency treatment of articular branches of femoral and obturator nerves for chronic hip pain. Clin Interv Aging 2015;10:569–74.

48. Cohen SP, Peterlin BL, Fulton L, et al. Randomized, double-blind, comparative-effectiveness study comparing pulsed radiofrequency to steroid injections for occipital neuralgia or migraine with occipital nerve tenderness. Pain 2015;156(12):2585–94.

49. Vanderhoek MD, Hoang HT, Goff B. Ultrasound-guided greater occipital nerve blocks and pulsed radiofrequency ablation for diagnosis and treatment of occipital neuralgia. Anesth Pain Med 2013;3(2): 256–9.

50. Vanelderen P, Rouwette T, De Vooght P, et al. Pulsed radiofrequency for the treatment of occipital neuralgia: a prospective study with 6 months of follow-up. Reg Anesth Pain Med 2010;35(2):148–51.

51. Colucci V, Strichartz G, Jolesz F, et al. Focused ultrasound effects on nerve action potential in vitro. Ultrasound Med Biol 2009;35(10):1737–47.

52. Dickey TC, Tych R, Kliot M, et al. Intense focused ultrasound can reliably induce sensations in human test subjects in a manner correlated with the density of their mechanoreceptors. Ultrasound Med Biol 2012;38(1):85–90.

53. Lee YF, Lin CC, Cheng JS, et al. High-intensity focused ultrasound attenuates neural responses of

sciatic nerves isolated from normal or neuropathic rats. Ultrasound Med Biol 2015;41(1):132–42.

54. Emril DR, Ho KY. Treatment of trigeminal neuralgia: role of radiofrequency ablation. J Pain Res 2010;3: 249–54.

55. Prabhala T, Hellman A, Walling I, et al. External focused ultrasound treatment for neuropathic pain induced by common peroneal nerve injury. Neurosci Lett 2018;684:145–51.

56. Walling I, Panse D, Gee L, et al. The use of focused ultrasound for the treatment of cutaneous allodynia associated with chronic migraine. Brain Res 2018; 1699:135–41.

57. Youn Y, Hellman A, Walling I, et al. High-Intensity Ultrasound Treatment for Vincristine-Induced Neuropathic Pain. Neurosurgery 2018;83(5):1068–75.

58. Hellman A, Maietta T, Byraju K, et al. Effects of external low intensity focused ultrasound on electrophysiological changes in vivo in a rodent model of common peroneal nerve injury. Neuroscience 2020;429:264–72.

59. Hellman A, Maietta T, Clum A, et al. Pilot study on the effects of low intensity focused ultrasound in a swine model of neuropathic pain. J Neurosurg 2021;1–8.

60. Masciocchi C, Zugaro L, Arrigoni F, et al. Radiofrequency ablation versus magnetic resonance guided focused ultrasound surgery for minimally invasive treatment of osteoid osteoma: a propensity score matching study. Eur Radiol 2016;26(8):2472–81.

61. Hellman A, Maietta T, Clum A, et al. Development of a common peroneal nerve injury model in domestic swine for the study of translational neuropathic pain treatments. J Neurosurg 2021;1–8.

62. Burgess A, Hynynen K. Drug delivery across the blood-brain barrier using focused ultrasound. Expert Opin Drug Deliv 2014;11(5):711–21.

63. McDannold N, Arvanitis CD, Vykhodtseva N, et al. Temporary disruption of the blood-brain barrier by use of ultrasound and microbubbles: safety and efficacy evaluation in rhesus macaques. Cancer Res 2012;72(14):3652–63.

64. Thévenot E, Jordão JF, O'Reilly MA, et al. Targeted delivery of self-complementary adeno-associated virus serotype 9 to the brain, using magnetic resonance imaging-guided focused ultrasound. Hum Gene Ther 2012;23(11):1144–55.

65. Payne AH, Hawryluk GW, Anzai Y, et al. Magnetic resonance imaging-guided focused ultrasound to increase localized blood-spinal cord barrier permeability. Neural Regen Res 2017;12(12):2045–9.

66. Mainprize T, Lipsman N, Huang Y, et al. Blood-Brain Barrier Opening in Primary Brain Tumors with Noninvasive MR-Guided Focused Ultrasound: A Clinical Safety and Feasibility Study. Sci Rep 2019;9(1):321.

67. Yang FY, Lin YS, Kang KH, et al. Reversible blood-brain barrier disruption by repeated transcranial focused ultrasound allows enhanced extravasation. J Control Release 2011;150(1):111–6.

68. Darrow DP. Focused Ultrasound for Neuromodulation. Neurotherapeutics 2019;16(1):88–99.

69. Airan RD, Meyer RA, Ellens NP, et al. Noninvasive Targeted Transcranial Neuromodulation via Focused Ultrasound Gated Drug Release from Nanoemulsions. Nano Lett 2017;17(2):652–9.

70. Wiffen PJ, Derry S, Bell RF, et al. Gabapentin for chronic neuropathic pain in adults. Cochrane Database Syst Rev 2017;6(6):Cd007938.

71. Quintero GC. Review about gabapentin misuse, interactions, contraindications and side effects. J Exp Pharmacol 2017;9:13–21.

72. Jung NY, Chang JW. Magnetic Resonance-Guided Focused Ultrasound in Neurosurgery: Taking Lessons from the Past to Inform the Future. J Korean Med Sci 2018;33(44):e279.

73. Hynynen K, McDannold N, Vykhodtseva N, et al. Noninvasive MR imaging-guided focal opening of the blood-brain barrier in rabbits. Radiology 2001; 220(3):640–6.

74. Tung YS, Marquet F, Teichert T, et al. Feasibility of noninvasive cavitation-guided blood-brain barrier opening using focused ultrasound and microbubbles in nonhuman primates. Appl Phys Lett 2011; 98(16):163704.

75. Marquet F, Tung YS, Teichert T, et al. Noninvasive, transient and selective blood-brain barrier opening in non-human primates in vivo. PLoS One 2011; 6(7):e22598.

76. Kovacs ZI, Kim S, Jikaria N, et al. Disrupting the blood-brain barrier by focused ultrasound induces sterile inflammation. Proc Natl Acad Sci U S A 2017;114(1):E75–84.

Ablation Procedures

Anthony Kaspa Allam, M. Benjamin Larkin Michael, MD, PharmD,
Ben Shofty, MD, PhD, Ashwin Viswanathan, MD*

KEYWORDS

- Ablation • Cancer pain • Cordotomy • Myelotomy • Cingulotomy

KEY POINTS

- Cordotomy is supported by level 2 evidence for unilateral cancer-related pain.
- Myelotomy is supported by level 3 evidence for visceral cancer pain.
- Cingulotomy may have use for widespread cancer pain with an affective component.
- Randomized controlled crossover trials demonstrating safety and efficacy will allow broader adoption of myelotomy, cingulotomy, and trigeminal tractotomy.

INTRODUCTION

Ablative surgery has little role in the management of chronic non-cancer-related pain, with the notable exception of trigeminal neuralgia. Targeted interventions such as percutaneous radiofrequency trigeminal gangliolysis, percutaneous balloon compression of the gasserian ganglion, and stereotactic radiosurgery are remarkably effective in controlling the triggerable, evoked pain of idiopathic trigeminal neuralgia.[1–8] However, for most other chronic pain states, ablative surgery has little evidence to support its use, and neuromodulation techniques including spinal cord stimulation, intrathecal drug delivery, dorsal root ganglion stimulation, and peripheral nerve stimulation have emerged as evidence-based treatment options for chronic pain.[9–13]

In the management of cancer-related pain, ablative surgery remains an essential treatment option.[9,14] A substantial portion of patients with active cancer can develop pain that is refractory to multimodal pharmacologic and nonpharmacologic treatment options.[15,16] Although intrathecal drug delivery is an evidence-based treatment option to reduce opioid-induced neurotoxicity, reduce pain, and perhaps improve survival in patients with cancer-related pain, there are several instances (structural pathologies, current chemotherapy treatment, expected survival, patient preference) in which this may not be an appropriate

intervention for a patient suffering from cancer-related pain.[17,18]

Ablative techniques have a few important advantages in the management of cancer-related pain. First, these techniques are often percutaneous or minimally invasive and hence can be performed at any stage of disease and during active cancer treatment. Second, these interventions confer an immediate benefit to the patient, without the need of titration of intrathecal therapy, and they require no ongoing maintenance. Finally, these interventions are useful especially for patients who are refractory to opioid therapy.[16,19–38] There are 4 interventions that are used with some frequency in the management of cancer-related pain, and they target the 4 types of pain that can arise in patients with cancer. In this review, cordotomy (spinothalamic tract ablation), myelotomy (dorsal columns visceral pain pathway ablation), and cingulotomy (cingulate gyrus ablation) are discussed. Trigeminal tractotomy (spinal trigeminal tract and nucleus ablation) is not discussed, although it is a useful intervention in the management of patients with head and neck malignancies and trigeminal neuropathic pain following craniotomy for skull base tumors.[5,39]

CORDOTOMY

Cordotomy is a lesion of the spinothalamic tract that carries somatic nociceptive sensation along

Department of Neurosurgery, Baylor College of Medicine, 7200 Cambridge Street, Suite 9A, Houston, TX 77030, USA
* Corresponding author.
E-mail address: ashwinv@bcm.edu

Neurosurg Clin N Am 33 (2022) 339–344
https://doi.org/10.1016/j.nec.2022.02.014

with other sensory modalities including temperature and itch.[40,41] Although cordotomy may have the best efficacy for patients with purely nociceptive pain, rarely is pain due to cancer purely nociceptive, and good results have been published for those patients with mixed nociceptive-neuropathic pain states.[30,31,34] Cordotomy will have variable effects on hot and cold perception thresholds, but this consequence is well tolerated because these sensations will be preserved in the contralateral body and in the nonlesioned portions of the spinothalamic tract.[40,42,43]

Several surgical techniques have been used for cordotomy. These include open thoracic cordotomy, open C1-C2 cordotomy, endoscopic C1-C2 cordotomy, fluoroscopically guided percutaneous C1-C2 cordotomy, and computed tomography (CT)-guided percutaneous C1-C2 cordotomy, which was introduced and popularized by Professor Kanpolat.[44] Of these modalities, CT-guided cordotomy has emerged as the dominant means for performing cordotomy. Although an open thoracic cordotomy may be considered for patients with bilateral cancer pain, it is a morbid procedure requiring a thoracic laminectomy and opening of the dura.[19] This procedure is often not appropriate for a patient who is toward the end of life and should be undertaken with caution in patients with impaired wound healing associated with systemic chemotherapy. In addition, anatomic tracing studies have clearly demonstrated that in the thoracic spine, some fibers of the spinothalamic tract reside dorsal to the dentate ligament.[40,45] Because lesions dorsal to the dentate ligament are not advisable due to the potential of injury to the corticospinal tract, bilateral open thoracic cordotomy carries the risk of persistent pain due to unlesioned fibers of the corticospinal tract.

Percutaneous CT-guided cordotomy is a safe intervention.[19,30–32,34,35,37,46] Even in patients with thrombocytopenia, who can be transfused to a platelet count of 50,000 to 75,000, the risk of bleeding within the spinal cord is low. Nonetheless, a careful informed consent discussion is needed when performing high cervical cordotomy in patients with platelet counts less than 100,000. It is not advisable to perform cordotomy without the use of intrathecal contrast. It is optimal to perform a lumbar puncture for the instillation of intrathecal contrast before procedure allowing time for distribution to the cervical spine.[44] The contrast provides excellent visualization of the spinal cord, which assists with the optimal placement of the radiofrequency electrode within the anterolateral quadrant of the spinal cord.[30,44] Although it may be possible on some CT scans to visualize the

cord without intrathecal contrast, it is a far inferior technique. However, if there are anatomic factors (multilevel tumor in the lumbar spine) or patient-related factors (inability to lie lateral or prone) that preclude lumbar puncture, contrast can also be instilled at the C1-C2 level.[44] In additional, the myelogram allows for the identification of an optimal entry point for the spinal needle before dural puncture.

Cordotomy is not a painful operation, and hence performing the procedure in the awake patient to allow intraoperative testing may optimize targeting of the intended portion of the spinothalamic tract, and minimize complications due to interruption of the corticospinal tract. A key principle of radiofrequency ablation is the ability to perform test stimulation before lesioning. In radiofrequency cordotomy, sensory stimulation is performed at a frequency of 100 Hz and a pulse width of 0.1 ms.[37,47] At an amplitude of less than 0.5 V, sensations are often elicited in the contralateral arm, trunk, or leg. The position of the radiofrequency electrode can be adjusted to target the painful region of the body. Generally, moving the electrode posteriorly and laterally can target the leg, whereas movement anteriorly or medially can target the arm.[48] There are patients in whom sensation cannot be elicited in the painful region of the body due to deafferentation. In this situation, if the operator can obtain stimulation in neighboring anatomic regions, cordotomy may still be successful. Another not uncommon finding is ipsilateral stimulation. This finding can occur for 3 reasons—an electrode that is contralateral to the needle insertion site, an electrode that is too dorsally placed, and from stimulation of uncrossed spinothalamic tract fibers.

Two lesions at 80°C for 60 seconds each in different locations within the anterolateral quadrant of the spinal cord is a generally accepted strategy used by those with some experience in this procedure.[19,30,34,37,46,48] Lower temperatures (ie, 70°C) and the use of one lesion may carry the risk of early pain recurrence or partial pain relief due to underlesioning the spinothalamic tract. In contrast, the use of 3 or 4 lesions likely carries the risk of unpleasant dysesthetic sensations, which can be as bothersome as the original pain for which the cordotomy was performed.[30]

MYELOTOMY

Refractory visceral pain, although less common in terms of presentation to the neurosurgeon, is another syndrome that is amenable to spinal cord ablation. Visceral pain is carried through the dorsal column's visceral pain pathway that ascends between the dorsal columns.[21,22,49] Similar to cordotomy, various surgical approaches have been used to perform myelotomy.[21,25,50] An open commissural myelotomy is a morbid procedure requiring a multilevel laminectomy and dural opening, which seeks to interrupt both the commissural fibers of the spinothalamic tract and the dorsal column's visceral pain pathway.[25,44] Percutaneous approaches targeting the visceral pain pathway have also been explored at the occipitocervical junction and thoracic spine using both radiofrequency and mechanical lesions to the spinal cord.[20,23,24,26,27,51–53] Probably most common today is an open thoracic laminectomy for lesioning of the visceral pain pathway. Although this procedure requires a single-level laminectomy and dural opening, it is reasonably well tolerated and may have better pain outcomes based on the limited case series published to date.[25,28,38,49]

Safe myelotomy is predicated on accurately identifying the midline of the spinal cord and creating an adequate lesion. Midline of the spinal cord is identified using multiple confirmatory techniques including intraoperative physiologic monitoring, observing the midpoint of the dorsal spinal rootlets, and localization of vasculature that penetrates the midline of the spinal cord. A mechanical lesion can be created with 1 mm width (0.5 mm on either side of the midline) and 1 mm craniocaudal extent. As with cordotomy, myelotomy interrupts an ascending pain pathway, and consequently, a long craniocaudal extent of the lesion is not needed. The main consideration is to lesion cephalad to where pain sensation from the affected part of the body enters the spinal cord. For pelvic pain, a lesion at T10 is appropriate, whereas for epigastric pain a more cephalad lesion at T3 is prudent.[22] Care must be exercised to avoid a lesion depth of greater than 5 mm to avoid injuring the anterior spinal artery.[28,29] One sequelae that is important to include in the informed consent discussion with the patient is the potential for disruption of the dorsal columns. Although this is a reasonably well-tolerated side effect, and an acceptable tradeoff for pain relief, interruption of the dorsal columns can lead to proprioceptive deficits, which can require physical therapy to ensure safe ambulation.

CINGULOTOMY

Although cordotomy and myelotomy are useful for relatively focal pain conditions, there is a population of patients with cancer-related pain with extensive bilateral pain, or pain that also has a substantial suffering component.[16] In these patients, spinal cord ablation is likely not to lead to meaningful pain improvement. Cingulotomy, or a bilateral lesion of the anterior cingulate gyrus, is a useful intervention to reduce pain and alleviate the suffering component associated with intractable cancer pain. Although our understanding of optimal patient selection for cingulotomy is still being developed, our knowledge of the optimal patients for spinal cord ablation and intrathecal drug delivery can guide identification of the optimal patient. Patients with unilateral cancer pain below the C5 dermatome should be treated with cordotomy. Patients with visceral pain will benefit from myelotomy. Patients who are opioid responsive, but with opioid-induced neurotoxicity, are likely excellent intrathecal pump candidates. Although experience with hypophysectomy for cancer pain is small, patients with widespread pain due to bony metastasis are likely best treated with radiosurgical hypophysectomy. For other complex pain conditions, with an affective component to the pain, cingulotomy should be considered. It is important in counseling patients, and equally importantly their families, to share that patients will likely experience some flattening of their affect postoperatively. Although this is a desired consequence of cingulotomy in the short term, because it reduces the anxiety that accompanies intractable pain, it can be a concerning finding to caregivers, and other treatment team members, if they do not know to expect this outcome.

There are 2 technical options for performing cingulotomy—radiofrequency ablation[54] and laser interstitial thermal therapy (LITT).[55] The advantage of radiofrequency cingulotomy is that it is a fast, inexpensive, and minimally invasive procedure that can be performed under minimal sedation if a patient cannot tolerate general anesthesia. Another critical advantage of radiofrequency cingulotomy is that 2 trajectories can easily be introduced if the surgeon prefers. LITT, in contrast, is likely a technique with which more functional neurosurgeons today have greater experience, given its widespread use in the treatment of neuro-oncology and epilepsy. Although LITT is a more expensive and time-consuming technique, it does confer the advantage of providing real-time feedback on the lesion size and geometry, and hence may be an advantageous technique for avoiding the subcortical U-fibers.

SUMMARY

Obtaining level 1 evidence for pain interventions in patients with cancer is challenging from both a feasibility perspective, and an ethical perspective.[56] Although there is a substantial placebo effect for pain interventions in noncancer patients, there is likely a much smaller placebo effect in patients suffering from cancer-related pain. Nonblinded, randomized controlled crossover trials of cancer pain interventions can provide substantial support for cancer pain interventions,[34] and are much more amenable to use in the patient with a short life expectancy due to cancer. Prospective series focusing on myelotomy, cingulotomy, and trigeminal tractotomy are keenly needed to allow these interventions to have broader adoption in the management of cancer-related pain.

CLINICS CARE POINTS

- When performing a cordotomy, two lesions at 80°C for 60 seconds each in different locations is considered the standard of treatment in order to minimize risk of pain recurrence and unpleasant dysesthesias.

- A common complication of a myelotomy includes the disruption of proprioceptive information in the dorsal column pathway. Patients must be advised of balance issues following the procedure.

- A cingulotomy affects the affective-emotional aspect of pain. As such, it is best advised for pain that is widespread, has a psychological component, and/or is located in the head/neck region.

DISCLOSURE

None.

REFERENCES

1. Skirving DJ, Dan NG. 20-year review of RFA TN. J Neurosurg 2001;94(6):913–7.
2. Kouzounias K, Schechtmann G, Lind G, et al. Factors that influence outcome of percutaneous balloon compression in the treatment of trigeminal neuralgia. Neurosurgery 2010;67(4):925–34.
3. Dhople AA, Adams JR, Maggio WW, et al. Longterm outcomes of Gamma Knife radiosurgery for classic trigeminal neuralgia: Implications of treatment and critical review of the literature - clinical article. J Neurosurg 2009;111(2):351–8.
4. Tuleasca C, Régis J, Sahgal A, et al. Stereotactic radiosurgery for trigeminal neuralgia: a systematic review. J Neurosurg 2019;130(3):733–57.
5. Reddy GD, Viswanathan A. Trigeminal and glossopharyngeal neuralgia. Neurol Clin 2014;32(2):539–52.
6. Park SS, Lee MK, Kim JW, et al. Percutaneous balloon compression of trigeminal ganglion for the treatment of idiopathic trigeminal neuralgia : experience in 50 patients. J Korean Neurosurg Soc 2008;43(4):186–9.
7. Kanpolat Y, Savas A, Bekar A, et al. Percutaneous controlled radiofrequency trigeminal rhizotomy for the treatment of idiopathic trigeminal neuralgia: 25-year experience with 1,600 patients. Neurosurgery 2001;48(3):524–32 [discussion: 532-4].
8. Taha JM, Tew JM, Buncher CR. A prospective 15-year follow up of 154 consecutive patients with trigeminal neuralgia treated by percutaneous stereotactic radiofrequency thermal rhizotomy. J Neurosurg 1995;83(6):989–93.
9. Franzini A, Moosa S, Servello D, et al. Ablative brain surgery: an overview. Int J Hyperthermia 2019;36(2):64–80.
10. North RB, Kidd DH, Zahurak M, et al. SNS in pain. Neurosurgery 1993;32(3):384–94 [discussion: 394-5].
11. Deer TR, Grigsby E, Weiner RL, et al. A prospective study of dorsal root ganglion stimulation for the relief of chronic pain. Neuromodulation 2013;16(1):67–72.
12. Xu J, Sun Z, Wu J, et al. Systematic Review Peripheral Nerve Stimulation in Pain Management: A Systematic Review. www.painphysicianjournal.
13. Amirdelfan K, Yu C, Doust MW, et al. Long-term quality of life improvement for chronic intractable back and leg pain patients using spinal cord stimulation: 12-month results from the SENZA-RCT. Qual Life Res 2018;27(8):2035–44.
14. Raslan AM, Ben-Haim S, Falowski SM, et al. Congress of neurological surgeons systematic review and evidence-based guideline on neuroablative procedures for patients with cancer pain. Neurosurgery 2021;88(3):437–42.
15. Lordon SP. Interventional Approach to Cancer Pain. Current Science Inc 2002;6:202–06.
16. Viswanathan A, Harsh V, Pereira EAC, et al. Cingulotomy for medically refractory cancer pain. Neurosurg Focus 2013;35(3).
17. Bhatia G, Lau ME, Gulur P. Intrathecal Drug Delivery (ITDD) systems for cancer pain. F1000Research 2013;2:96.
18. Stearns LM, Abd-Elsayed A, Perruchoud C, et al. Intrathecal drug delivery systems for cancer pain: An analysis of a prospective, multicenter product surveillance registry. Anesth Analgesia 2020;289–97.
19. Javed S, Viswanathan A, Abdi S. Cordotomy for Intractable Cancer Pain: A Narrative Review. Pain physician 2020;23(3):283–92. Available at: http://www.ncbi.nlm.nih.gov/pubmed/32517394.
20. Vilela Filho O, Araujo MR, Florencio RS, et al. CT-guided percutaneous punctate midline myelotomy for the treatment of intractable visceral pain: a

technical note. Stereotactic Funct Neurosurg 2001; 77(1–4):177–82.

21. Nauta HJW, Westlund KN, WW. Midline myelotomy and the interruption of the postsynaptic dorsal column path-way for the treatment of visceral pain. In: Burchiel KJ, editor. Handbook of pain surgery. Thieme; 2018. p. 312–33.

22. Willis WD, Al-Chaer ED, Quast MJ, et al. A visceral pain pathway in the dorsal column of the spinal cord. Proc Natl Acad Sci 1999;96(14):7675–9.

23. Gildenberg PL, Hirshberg RM. Limited myelotomy for the treatment of intractable cancer pain. J Neurol Neurosurg Psychiatry 1984;47(1):94–6.

24. Nauta HJW, Soukup VM, Fabian RH, et al. Punctate midline myelotomy for the relief of visceral cancer pain. J Neurosurg Spine 2000;92(2):125–30.

25. Viswanathan A, Burton AW, Rekito A, et al. Commissural myelotomy in the treatment of intractable visceral pain: technique and outcomes. Stereotactic Funct Neurosurg 2010;88(6):374–82.

26. Schvarcz JR. Stereotactic extralemniscal myelotomy. J Neurol Neurosurg Psychiatry 1976;39(1):53–7.

27. Eiras J, Garcia J, Gomez J, et al. First results with extralemniscal myelotomy. In: ; 1980:377-381.

28. Vedantam A, Koyyalagunta D, Bruel BM, et al. Limited midline myelotomy for intractable visceral pain: surgical techniques and outcomes. Neurosurgery 2018;83(4):783–9.

29. Larkin MB, North RY, Vedantam A, et al. Limited midline myelotomy for visceral pain. Neurosurg Focus: Video 2020;3(2):V16.

30. Kanpolat Y, Ugur HC, Ayten M, et al. Computed tomography-guided percutaneous cordotomy for intractable pain in malignancy. Neurosurgery 2009; 64(3 Suppl):ons187–93 [discussion: ons193-4].

31. Raslan AM. Percutaneous computed tomography-guided radiofrequency ablation of upper spinal cord pain pathways for cancer-related pain. Neurosurgery 2008;62(3 Suppl 1):226–33 [discussion: 233-4].

32. Raslan AM, Cetas JS, Mccartney S, et al. Destructive procedures for control of cancer pain: The case for cordotomy: A review. J Neurosurg 2011; 114(1):155–70.

33. Larkin MB, Karas PJ, McGinnis JP, et al. Stereotactic radiosurgery hypophysectomy for palliative treatment of refractory cancer pain: a historical review and update. Front Oncol 2020;10. https://doi.org/10.3389/fonc.2020.572557.

34. Viswanathan A, Vedantam A, Hess KR, et al. Minimally invasive cordotomy for refractory cancer pain: a randomized controlled trial. The Oncologist 2019;24(7):e590–6.

35. Reddy GD, Okhuysen-Cawley R, Harsh V, et al. Percutaneous CT-guided cordotomy for the treatment of pediatric cancer pain. J Neurosurg Pediatr 2013;12(1):93–6.

36. Gadgil N, Viswanathan A. DREZotomy in the treatment of cancer pain: A review. Stereotactic Funct Neurosurg 2012;90(6):356–60.

37. Strauss I, Berger A, Arad M, et al. O-arm-guided percutaneous radiofrequency cordotomy. Stereotactic Funct Neurosurg 2018;95(6):409–16.

38. Ball T, Aljuboori Z, Nauta H. Midthoracic punctate midline myelotomy for treatment of chronic, intractable, nonmalignant, abdominal visceral pain: 2-dimensional operative video. Oper Neurosurg 2020;19(2):E183.

39. Larkin MB, North RY, Viswanathan A. Percutaneous computed tomography-guided radiofrequency ablation of spinal trigeminal tract and nucleus caudalis for refractory trigeminal neuropathic pain: 2-dimensional operative video. Oper Neurosurg 2020; 19(5):E530–1.

40. Vedantam A, Bruera E, Hess KR, et al. Somatotopy and organization of spinothalamic tracts in the human cervical spinal cord. Neurosurgery 2019; 84(6):E311–7.

41. Taren JA, Davis R, Crosby EC. Target physiologic corroboration in stereotaxic cervical cordotomy. J Neurosurg 1969;30(5):569–84.

42. Lahuerta J, Bowsher D, Campbell J, et al. Clinical and instrumental evaluation of sensory function before and after percutaneous anterolateral cordotomy at cervical level in man. Pain 1990;42(1):23–30.

43. Friehs GM, Schröttner O, Pendl G. Evidence for segregated pain and temperature conduction within the spinothalamic tract. J Neurosurg 1995;83(1):8–12.

44. Kanpolat Y. The surgical treatment of chronic pain: Destructive therapies in the spinal cord. Neurosurg Clin North America 2004;15(3):307–17.

45. Zhang X, Honda CN, Giesler GJ. Position of spinothalamic tract axons in upper cervical spinal cord of monkeys. J Neurophysiol 2000;84(3):1180–5.

46. Larkin MB, North RY, Viswanathan A. Percutaneous CT-guided cordotomy for pain. Neurosurg Focus: Video 2020;3(2):V15.

47. Vedantam A, Hou P, Chi TL, et al. Postoperative MRI evaluation of a radiofrequency cordotomy lesion for intractable cancer pain. AJNR Am J neuroradiology 2017;38(4):835–9.

48. Shepherd TM, Hoch MJ, Cohen BA, et al. Palliative CT-Guided cordotomy for medically intractable pain in patients with cancer. Am J Neuroradiology 2017;38(2):387–90.

49. Nauta HJ, Hewitt E, Westlund KN, et al. Surgical interruption of a midline dorsal column visceral pain pathway. Case report and review of the literature. J Neurosurg 1997;86(3):538–42.

50. Raslan AM, Burchiel KJ. Neurosurgical Advances in Cancer Pain Management. Curr Pain Headache Rep 2010;14(6):477–82.

51. Kim YS, Kwon SJ. High thoracic midline dorsal column myelotomy for severe visceral pain due to

advanced stomach cancer. Neurosurgery 2000; 46(1):85–90 [discussion: 90-2]. Available at: http://www.ncbi.nlm.nih.gov/pubmed/10626939.

52. Hwang SL, Lin CL, Lieu AS, et al. Punctate midline myelotomy for intractable visceral pain caused by hepatobiliary or pancreatic cancer. J Pain Symptom Manage 2004;27(1):79–84.

53. North RB, Lanning A, Hessels R, et al. Spinal cord stimulation with percutaneous and plate electrodes: side effects and quantitative comparisons. Neurosurg Focus 1997;2(1):E5.

54. Patel NV, Agarwal N, Mammis A, et al. Frameless stereotactic magnetic resonance imaging-guided laser interstitial thermal therapy to perform bilateral anterior cingulotomy for intractable pain: feasibility, technical aspects, and initial experience in 3 patients. Oper Neurosurg (Hagerstown) 2015;(Suppl 2):17–25 [discussion: 25].

55. Strauss I, Berger A, Ben Moshe S, et al. Double anterior stereotactic cingulotomy for intractable oncological pain. Stereotact Funct Neurosurg 2017;95(6):400–8.

56. Viswanathan A, Vedantam A, Williams LA, et al. Percutaneous cordotomy for pain palliation in advanced cancer: a randomized clinical trial study protocol. Neurosurgery 2020;87(2):394–402.

Imaging as a Pain Biomarker

Alon Kashanian, MD[a,1], Evangelia Tsolaki, PhD[b], James Caruso, MD[c,2], Ausaf Bari, MD, PhD[b], Nader Pouratian, MD, PhD[c,*]

KEYWORDS

- Biomarker ● Chronic pain ● Diffusion ● DTI ● Functional ● fMRI ● Imaging ● MRI

KEY POINTS

- Anatomic, diffusion, and functional imaging studies demonstrate various measurable brain alterations, which may signify pain biomarkers for several chronic pain disorders.
- Biomarkers of interest include areas within somatosensory pain processing regions as well as brain regions involved in mediating affective and cognitive processes in certain chronic pain disorders.
- A multimodal approach that integrates radiological, behavioral, physiologic, and omics measures may provide the most robust objective method for pain assessment.
- Most evidence in support of radiological pain biomarkers is derived from studies conducted in a research setting. Clinical application and controlled trials are lacking.

INTRODUCTION

Chronic pain is one of the most prevalent and critical public health problems in the United States and globally. According to the Centers for Disease Control and Prevention, chronic pain affects approximately 50 million US adults[1] and costs more than $560 to 635 billion each year, nearly 30% higher than the combined cost of cancer and diabetes.[2] Given that each day in the United States more than 90 individuals die from opioid overdose,[3] identifying effective nonopioid therapies for the treatment of chronic pain is a top health care priority. In recent years, the hunt for objective biomarkers in chronic pain has intensified as interest has grown in precision medicine techniques and the global opioid crisis has underscored the need to accelerate the pace of pain research.[4]

However, there remain no objective, measurable biomarkers to explain the diversity in response to established treatments for chronic pain. A growing body of neuroimaging literature suggests that chronic pain is associated with various alterations in regional brain areas as well as whole-brain networks, which may represent unique radiological pain signatures or biomarkers to guide diagnosis, response, and treatment.[5] To this end we provide a comprehensive and updated literature review on investigative efforts to identify neuroimaging biomarkers for pain.

ANATOMIC IMAGING

The search for pain biomarkers has motivated several neuroanatomic imaging studies, which have demonstrated that altered brain morphology frequently accompanies chronic pain conditions. Structural changes in gray matter (GM) were first reported in patients with chronic back pain (CBP)[6,7] and have since been shown in many other chronic pain conditions such as complex regional

[a] Department of Surgery, Donald and Barbara Zucker School of Medicine, Hofstra/Northwell, Manhasset, NY, USA; [b] Department of Neurosurgery, University of California Los Angeles, 300 Stein Plaza, Suite 562, Los Angeles, CA 90095, USA; [c] Department of Neurological Surgery, University of Texas Southwestern, Dallas, TX, USA

[1] Present address: 350 Community Drive, Manhasset, NY 11030.
[2] Present address: 5303 Harry Hines Boulevard, 6th Floor, Dallas, TX 75390.
* Corresponding author. 5323 Harry Hines Boulevard, MC 8855, Dallas, TX 75390.
E-mail address: nader.pouratian@utsouthwestern.edu
Twitter: @AlonKashanian (A.K.); @Evie_Tsolaki (E.T.); @ausaf (A.B.); @drpouratian (N.P.)

Neurosurg Clin N Am 33 (2022) 345–350
https://doi.org/10.1016/j.nec.2022.02.011

pain syndrome (CRPS),[8] fibromyalgia,[9] osteoarthritis (OA),[10] irritable bowel syndrome (IBS),[11] migraine,[12] and several others.[13] Generally, when compared with healthy controls, patients with chronic pain display regional decreases in GM in areas typically associated with pain, such as the anterior cingulate cortex, insula, and thalamus, although no change or increased GM volume has also been reported in some regions such as the hippocampus and parahippocampal gyrus.[14] Although many studies emphasize the involvement of brain regions in the "pain matrix," the data also suggest changes in brain areas that are not commonly associated with pain processing, and that unique brain regions are impacted in different types of chronic pain.[14] Baliki and colleagues[13] evaluated changes in brain structure using MRI in patients suffering from CBP, CRPS, and knee OA relative to healthy controls. The investigators parceled the brain into 82 brain regions and generated a structural covariance to map anatomic interrelationships within the cortex for each group. The investigators found substantial brain anatomic reorganization specific to each condition and were able to robustly classify individuals to their respective grouping by using the 82-region parcellation to generate a barcode. More recently, Qiu and colleagues[15] were able to detect differences in brain structure even between 2 types of peripheral neuropathic pain (postherpetic neuralgia and chronic low back pain [CLBP]), based on GM volume and morphologic connectivity. Novel multivariate machine learning approaches have played a valuable role in characterizing pain biomarkers in the field of structural imaging.[16,17] Ung and colleagues[16] extracted brain GM density from MRI scans of 47 patients with CLBP and 47 healthy controls, and were able to classify CLBP with an accuracy of 76% by using a support vector machine (SVM). Primary drivers of the classification included areas of the somatosensory, motor, and prefrontal cortices. Similar machine learning techniques have also shown utility for identifying meaningful neurobiological markers in chronic visceral pain disorders.[11,17] Bagarinao and colleagues[17] used a multivariate classification approach to detect changes in brain morphology associated with chronic pelvic pain (CPP) and to identify patterns to distinguish individuals with CPP from age-matched healthy controls. Regions of positive SVM weight included several regions within the primary somatosensory cortex (S1), left pre-supplementary motor area (pre-SMA), bilateral hippocampus, and left amygdala, which were identified as important drivers of the classification with 73% overall accuracy. In addition to distinguishing between patients with chronic pain and healthy controls, observed cerebral morphologic differences in chronic pain conditions often correlate to the number of years of pain individuals have been suffering with the condition as well as its intensity or frequency.[6,8,12] Using advanced MRI morphometry-based machine learning algorithms, patients with chronic migraine were distinguished from those with episodic migraine with 84.2% accuracy and from healthy controls with 86.3% accuracy.[12] The classifiers contained principal components consisting of several structural measures like the temporal pole, anterior cingulate cortex (ACC), superior temporal lobe, entorhinal cortex, medial orbital frontal gyrus, and pars triangularis. Finally, the significance of these biomarkers is further supported by studies that have demonstrated that many of the gray matter changes observed in patients with pain subside with cessation of pain.[10,18] Rodriguez-Raecke and Niemeier[10] investigated 32 patients with chronic pain due to primary hip OA and found a characteristic gray matter decrease in patients compared with controls in the ACC, right insular cortex and operculum, dorsolateral prefrontal cortex (DLPFC), amygdala, and brainstem. Within a subgroup of 10 patients who underwent total hip replacement surgery and were subsequently completely pain free, all had a gray matter increase in the DLPFC, ACC, amygdala, and brainstem after surgery. In total, the data suggest the presence of unique brain signatures or structural biomarkers for different pain disorders. However, future studies are needed to further improve classification and to assess whether the observed differences in brain structure are unique to specific pain conditions or generalizable to other chronic pain conditions.

MAGNETIC RESONANCE DIFFUSION IMAGING

In addition to anatomic morphometric studies, diffusion tensor imaging (DTI) has elucidated central and peripheral pain processing pathways that may serve as important diagnostic biomarkers for a range of pain disorders.

Much of the work in this area of neuroimaging has been used to classify patients with trigeminal neuralgia (TN) from healthy controls.[19,20] Zhang and colleagues[19] observed significant fractional anisotropy (FA) reductions and increased diffusivity at the affected trigeminal root entry zone and that these DTI-derived metrics were discriminating features for patients with TN according to an SVM approach. The investigators found that 1 week after effective treatment, diffusion recovery was mainly due to a decrease in parallel diffusivity, which is consistent with axonal membrane stabilization, whereas at 4 to 6 months it was due to a predominant reduction in perpendicular diffusivity, corresponding with remyelination. Zhong and colleagues[20] further showed that whole-brain tractography in combination with SVM algorithm could successfully differentiate patients with TN from healthy controls with 88% accuracy. Patients with TN were characterized by reduced fiber connections between regions related to affective and associative dimensions of pain and enhanced fiber connections of regions related to both somatosensory and higher-order cognitive functions. Szabó and colleagues[21] found that when compared with healthy controls, patients with migraine showed reduced FA, as well as increased radial and mean diffusivity (MD) in the right frontal white matter. The connectivity of the affected fiber bundle was similar to the pain network that includes periaqueductal gray (PAG) and cuneiform nucleus, prefrontal cortex, amygdala, thalamus and hypothalamus, and rostroventral medulla as was previously described by Hadjipavlou and colleagues.[22] In yet another study, voxelwise DTI and track density imaging were used to investigate the microstructural brain differences between patients with urologic chronic pelvic pain syndrome (UCPPS), IBS, and healthy controls.[23] The investigators found that patients with UCPPS showed elevated MD, lowered FA and generalized anisotropy, and lowered fiber track density compared with healthy controls in regions of the brain involved in supraspinal sensory processing including cingulate gyrus, temporal lobes, somatosensory integration areas, and frontal/prefrontal cortical projections. Results also showed significant differences in specific anatomic regions in patients with UCPPS when compared with patients with IBS, consistent with microstructural alterations specific to UCPPS.

DTI has also shown promise in identifying prognostic biomarkers and in discriminating treatment responders from nonresponders in individuals with chronic pain. Two longitudinal studies found that patients with CLBP had higher FA in the white matter (WM) of the left insula after treatment,[24] and that a greater frequency of WM connections within the dorsomedial prefrontal cortex-amygdala-nucleus accumbens circuit was an independent risk factor for pain persistence.[25] Diffusivity abnormalities in brainstem trigeminal fibers were helpful in a priori prediction of surgical nonresponders in a neurosurgical study of 31 patients with primary TN.[26] The study revealed 3 ipsilateral diffusivity thresholds of response—pontine axial diffusivity, MD, and cisternal FA—separating 85% of nonresponders from responders. Furthermore, in patients who underwent gamma-knife surgery to treat TN, postsurgical FA values were used to predict the level of pain relief 6 months after surgery.[27] Specifically, responders presented lower FA and achieved at least 75% reduction in pain, whereas nonresponders did not show the same decrease in diffusion metrics. Tractography-based deep brain stimulation for chronic pain disorders has already demonstrated benefit in guiding targeting and optimizing treatment outcomes.[28] Additional research in the field of DTI will be valuable for guiding further therapeutic intervention for chronic pain.

FUNCTIONAL IMAGING

Functional neuroimaging techniques, such as positron emission tomography and more recently functional MRI (fMRI), have provided unique insight into the central changes that occur with pain and have helped us visualize how these areas change over time. These imaging modalities suggest a more dynamic and interdependent conception of pain that is a result of multiple brain areas and networks rather than a localized view where the sensation of pain is pinpointed to a single site of injury or pathway. Moreover, these imaging studies have provided radiological evidence in support of the theory that pain is not solely a sensory process but a multidimensional one including affective and cognitive components. A meta-analysis of 152 studies that included individuals with acute and chronic pain found consistent activation across studies in several brain regions commonly referred to as the "pain matrix" that are in parallel with the 3 dimensions of pain.[29,30] These brain regions include S1 and secondary (S2) somatosensory cortices, insula, ACC, nucleus accumbens, amygdala, medial prefrontal cortex, and thalamus.[29] Wager and colleagues[31] conducted 4 different studies to determine an fMRI-based neurologic signature that could be used to quantify pain objectively. The investigators identified a universal pattern of fMRI activity, including the thalamus, the posterior and anterior insulae, S2, ACC, and PAG matter, that was associated with heat-induced pain to the forearm. This brain signature was not only able to differentiate between painful heat and nonpainful warmth with a sensitivity and specificity of 94% but was also able to discriminate between relative differences in pain with a sensitivity and specificity of 93%, with pain ratings differing by 2 or more points on a 9-point visual analog scale. Moreover, the strength of the signature response was substantially reduced when an analgesic agent, remifentanil, was administered.

Resting-state fMRI studies suggest alterations in large-scale brain networks, particularly the default mode network (DMN), may differentiate different types of chronic pain.[32,33] Loggia and colleagues[34] compared DMN connectivity between patients with CLBP and controls following physical maneuvers. At baseline, patients showed stronger DMN connectivity to the insula and less to the pregenual ACC. After physical maneuvers, an increase in low back pain was associated with an increase in DMN right insula connectivity. In their clinical investigation of the effect of ketamine for pain relief in patients with refractory neuropathic pain, Bosma and colleagues[35] found that pretreatment dynamic functional connectivity between the DMN and the descending antinociception pathway was associated with treatment effect. In addition, temporal summation of pain was significantly related to the dynamic functional connectivity between the DMN and descending antinociception pathway dynamic functional connectivity.[35]

Interestingly, several longitudinal studies have shown that as pain transitions from an acute to chronic state, there is shift away from somatosensory representation toward increased prominence of brain regions and pathways that mediate affective and cognitive processes.[32] For example, in their fMRI study, Hashmi and colleagues[36] found that whereas brain activity for those with acute or subacute back pain was limited to regions involved in acute pain, such as the insula, activity in patients with CBP was confined to structures involved in emotion-related circuitry, such as the medial prefrontal cortex. In fact, there is substantial evidence in the functional neuroimaging literature demonstrating overlap of activation in brain areas in individuals with depression and chronic pain.[37] This finding is further corroborated by statistics showing that patients with chronic pain display a higher incidence of comorbid psychiatric disorders such as depression, anxiety, and substance abuse.[38–40] Together, the evidence suggests that brain areas involved in emotional processing may serve as potential biomarkers and neuromodulatory targets for chronic pain.[37]

CHALLENGES AND OPPORTUNITIES

We provide a comprehensive and updated review of the literature investigating imaging as a pain biomarker. As described earlier, there is a significant amount of evidence to support the potential use of imaging as diagnostic, prognostic, or treatment-response biomarkers for clinical pain. Despite this, the application of these findings to clinical practice may be limited due to concern regarding the specificity of neuroimaging for pain measurement.[41] The concern stems from the

observation that almost identical functional neuroimaging response in areas of the "pain matrix" can be produced by nonpainful stimuli, therefore suggesting that these brain responses may not be specific for pain.[42] For example, Salomons and colleagues[43] demonstrated that they were able to elicit pain matrix responses on fMRI even in individuals who were congenitally unable to experience pain. Almost all the aforementioned studies in this review were conducted in a research setting. Furthermore, there are theoretic, philosophic, and measurement-based limitations of using neuroimaging to diagnose individuals with pain from those without, and these should be wholly considered before substituting radiological markers for self-report measures of pain.[9] Thus, caution should be taken in using pain matrix responses for diagnosis or drug discovery and highlight the need for studies with more carefully designed and rigorously tested controlled conditions.

Our review focuses primarily on the most common neuroimaging techniques, particularly brain imaging techniques, because these have been the most studied. However, this is not to minimize the importance of structural imaging of the spinal cord and peripheral tissues. Recent studies of spinal cord DTI demonstrate its nascent potential in assessing severity of spinal cord injury (SCI) and predicting postinjury neurologic outcomes.[44,45] With further development and clinical application, these techniques may prove useful for clarifying mechanisms of post-SCI neuropathic pain generation and identifying therapeutic targets. Moreover, novel noninvasive imaging methods for pain such as magnetic resonance (MR) elastography for assessing mechanical properties of tissue[46] and MR spectroscopy to quantify cellular and biochemical changes in the brain, blood, and other tissues, provide additional methods to objectify pain. Ultimately, a composite or multimodal approach that integrates radiological, behavioral, physiologic, and omics measures may provide the most robust objective pain assessment. The incorporation of machine learning algorithms could further enhance the specificity and accuracy of this assessment. Finally, the revelation of biomarkers has the potential to elucidate new pain targets and treatment strategies, which in turn have the potential to further reveal underlying mechanisms behind pathologic pain disorders.

SUMMARY

Anatomic, diffusion, and functional imaging studies demonstrate various measurable brain alterations, which may signify pain biomarkers for several chronic pain disorders. Biomarkers of interest include areas within somatosensory pain processing regions as well as brain regions involved in mediating affective and cognitive processes in certain chronic pain disorders. A composite or multimodal approach that integrates radiological, behavioral, physiologic, and omics measures may provide the most robust objective method for pain assessment. Evidence in support of radiological pain biomarkers is derived from studies conducted in a research setting. Future controlled clinical trials are required to validate these findings.

CLINICS CARE POINTS

- Chronic pain, even when related to peripheral etiologies, is likely related to changes in brain structure and function.
- Effective treatments may require consideration of novel approaches to central neuromodulation, but will likely vary on the type and etiology of pain.

ACKNOWLEDGEMENTS

This work is supported, in part, by funding from the National Institute of Neurological Disorders and Stroke UH3 NS113661.

DISCLOSURE

Dr N. Pouratian is a consultant for Abbott Laboratories.

REFERENCES

1. Dahlhamer JM, Lucas J, Zelaya C, et al. Prevalence of chronic pain and high-impact chronic pain among adults — United States, 2016. Morb Mortal Wkly Rep 2018;67(36):1001–6.
2. Gaskin DJ, Richard P. The economic costs of pain in the United States. J Pain 2012;13(8):715–24.
3. Wakeman SE. Facing Addiction. Psychiatric Annals 2019;49(2).
4. Davis KD, Aghaeepour N, Ahn AH, et al. Discovery and validation of biomarkers to aid the development of safe and effective pain therapeutics: challenges and opportunities. Nat Rev Neurol 2020;16(7):381.
5. Xu X, Huang Y. Objective pain assessment: a key for the management of chronic pain. F1000Research 2020;9.
6. Apkarian AV. Chronic back pain is associated with decreased prefrontal and thalamic gray matter density. J Neurosci 2004;24(46):10410–5.
7. Schmidt-Wilcke T, Leinisch E, Gänßbauer S, et al. Affective components and intensity of pain correlate with structural differences in gray matter in chronic back pain patients. Pain 2006;125(1–2):89–97.
8. Geha PY, Baliki MN, Harden RN, et al. The Brain in Chronic CRPS pain: abnormal gray-white matter interactions in emotional and autonomic regions. Neuron 2008;60(4):570–81.
9. Robinson ME, O'Shea AM, Craggs JG, et al. Comparison of Machine Classification Algorithms for Fibromyalgia: Neuroimages Versus Self-Report. J Pain 2015;16(5):472–7.
10. Rodriguez-Raecke R, Niemeier A. Ihle Kristin., et al. Brain Gray Matter Decrease in Chronic Pain Is the Consequence and Not the Cause of Pain. J Neurosci 2009;29(44):13746–50.
11. Labus JS, Van Horn JD, Gupta A, et al. Multivariate morphological brain signatures predict patients with chronic abdominal pain from healthy control subjects. Pain 2015;156(8):1545–54.
12. Schwedt TJ, Chong CD, Wu T, et al. Accurate classification of chronic migraine via brain magnetic resonance imaging. Headache J Head Face Pain 2015;55(6):762–77.
13. Baliki MN, Schnitzer TJ, Bauer WR, et al. Brain morphological signatures for chronic pain. PLoS One 2011;6(10):e26010.
14. Smallwood Rachel F, Laird Angela R, Ramage Amy E, et al. Structural brain anomalies and chronic pain: a quantitative meta-analysis of gray matter volume. J Pain 2013;14(7):663–75.
15. Qiu J, Du M, Yang J, et al. The brain's structural differences between postherpetic neuralgia and lower back pain. Sci Rep 2021 Nov 17;11(1):22455.
16. Ung H, Brown JE, Johnson Kevin A, et al. Multivariate classification of structural MRI data detects chronic low back pain. Cereb Cortex 2014;24(4):1037–44.
17. Bagarinao E, Johnson KA, Martucci KT, et al. Preliminary structural MRI based brain classification of chronic pelvic pain: a MAPP network study. Pain 2014;155(12):2502–9.
18. Obermann M, Nebel K, Schumann C, et al. Gray matter changes related to chronic posttraumatic headache. Neurology 2009;73(12):978–83.
19. Zhang Y, Mao Z, Cui Z, et al. Diffusion tensor imaging of axonal and myelin changes in classical trigeminal neuralgia. World Neurosurg 2018;112:e597–607.
20. Zhong J, Chen DQ, Hung PS, et al. Multivariate pattern classification of brain white matter connectivity predicts classic trigeminal neuralgia. Pain 2018;159(10):2076–87.
21. Szabó N, Kincses ZT, Párdutz Á, et al. White matter microstructural alterations in migraine: a diffusion-weighted MRI study. Pain 2012;153(3):651–6.

22. Hadjipavlou G, Dunckley P, Behrens TE, et al. Determining anatomical connectivities between cortical and brainstem pain processing regions in humans: a diffusion tensor imaging study in healthy controls. Pain 2006;123(1–2):169–78.

23. Woodworth D, Mayer E, Leu K, et al. Unique microstructural changes in the brain associated with urological chronic pelvic pain syndrome (UCPPS) revealed by diffusion tensor MRI, super-resolution track Density imaging, and statistical parameter mapping: a MAPP Network Neuroimaging Study. PLoS One 2015;10(10):e0140250.

24. Ceko M, Shir Y, Ouellet JA, et al. Partial recovery of abnormal insula and dorsolateral prefrontal connectivity to cognitive networks in chronic low back pain after treatment. Hum Brain Mapp 2015;36(6): 2075–92.

25. Vachon-Presseau E, Tétreault P, Petre B, et al. Corticolimbic anatomical characteristics predetermine risk for chronic pain. Brain 2016;139(7):1958–70.

26. Hung Peter S-P, Chen David Q, Davis Karen D, et al. Predicting pain relief: Use of pre-surgical trigeminal nerve diffusion metrics in trigeminal neuralgia. Neuroimage Clin 2017;15:710–8.

27. Tohyama S, Hung PS, Zhong J, et al. Early postsurgical diffusivity metrics for prognostication of long-term pain relief after Gamma Knife radiosurgery for trigeminal neuralgia. J Neurosurg JNS 2019;131(2): 539–48.

28. Kim TS, Park JY. Diffusion Tensor Imaging MRI for Chronic Pain Management. Asian J Pain 2016;2(1): 1–5.

29. May A. Neuroimaging: visualising the brain in pain. Neurol Sci 2007;28(Suppl 2):S101–7.

30. Peyron R, Laurent B, García-Larrea L. Functional imaging of brain responses to pain. A review and meta-analysis (2000). Neurophysiol Clin 2000; 30(5):263–88.

31. Wager TD, Atlas LY, Lindquist MA, et al. An fMRI-based neurologic signature of physical pain. N Engl J Med 2013;368(15):1388–97.

32. Ng SK, Urquhart DM, Fitzgerald PB, et al. The relationship between structural and functional brain changes and altered emotion and cognition in chronic low back pain brain changes: a systematic review of MRI and fMRI studies. Clin J Pain 2018; 34(3):237–61.

33. Kregel J, Meeus M, Malfliet A, et al. Structural and functional brain abnormalities in chronic low back pain: a systematic review. Semin Arthritis Rheum 2015;45(2):229–37.

34. Loggia ML, Kim J, Gollub RL, et al. Default mode network connectivity encodes clinical pain: An arterial spin labeling study. Pain 2013;154(1):24–33.

35. Bosma RL, Cheng JC, Rogachov A, et al. Brain dynamics and temporal summation of pain predicts neuropathic pain relief from ketamine infusion. Anesthesiology 2018;129(5):1015–24.

36. Hashmi JA, Baliki MN, Huang L, et al. Shape shifting pain: Chronification of back pain shifts brain representation from nociceptive to emotional circuits. Brain 2013;136(9):2751–68.

37. Kashanian A, Tsolaki E, Pouratian N, et al. Deep brain stimulation of the subgenual cingulate cortex for the treatment of chronic low back pain. Neuromodulation 2022;25(2):202–10.

38. Barry DT, Pilver CE, Hoff RA, et al. Pain interference and incident mood, anxiety, and substance-use disorders: findings from a representative sample of men and women in the general population. J Psychiatr Res 2013;47(11):1658–64.

39. Barry DT, Pilver C, Potenza MN, et al. Prevalence and psychiatric correlates of pain interference among men and women in the general population. J Psychiatr Res 2012;46(1):118–27.

40. Bair MJ, Robinson RL, Katon W, et al. Depression and pain comorbidity: a literature review. Arch Intern Med 2003;2433–45.

41. Mouraux A, Iannetti GD. The search for pain biomarkers in the human brain. Brain 2018;141(12): 3290–307.

42. Iannetti GD, Salomons TV, Moayedi M, et al. Beyond metaphor: contrasting mechanisms of social and physical pain. Trends Cogn Sci 2013;17(8):371–8.

43. Salomons TV, Iannetti GD, Liang M, et al. The "pain matrix" in pain-free individuals. JAMA Neurol 2016; 73(6):755–6.

44. Zaninovich OA, Avila MJ, Kay M, et al. The role of diffusion tensor imaging in the diagnosis, prognosis, and assessment of recovery and treatment of spinal cord injury: a systematic review. Neurosurg Focus 2019;46(3):E7.

45. Saksena Sona, Mohamed FB, Middleton DM, et al. Diffusion tensor imaging assessment of regional white matter changes in the cervical and thoracic spinal cord in pediatric subjects. J Neurotrauma 2019;36(6):853–61.

46. Chan DD, Cai L, Butz KD, et al. In vivo articular cartilage deformation: noninvasive quantification of intra-tissue strain during joint contact in the human knee. Sci Rep 2016;6:19220.

Machine Learning and Pain Outcomes

Tessa Harland, MD[a], Amir Hadanny, MD[a], Julie G. Pilitsis, MD, PhD[a,b,*]

KEYWORDS

• Machine learning • Pain outcomes • Pain management • Biomarker • Prediction • Patient selection

KEY POINTS

• Successful outcomes of a pain management intervention are largely dependent on appropriate patient selection; however, patients' different pain phenotypes have yet to be well-identified.
• Machine learning (ML) is a useful technique to develop algorithms that can predict which patients may benefit specific therapies.
• ML and its ability to formulate patterns and classify large amounts of complex data are a promising means to identify different pain phenotypes associated with positive and negative outcomes.

DEFINITIONS

• Artificial intelligence: the broader term which describes technologies that can perform tasks that typically require human intelligence.
• Machine learning (ML): a developing subfield of artificial intelligence in which computers learn from past data by automatically detecting patterns and using those patterns to develop algorithms that can be used to address future data.
• Supervised learning: a subdivision of ML that requires labeled data that is already marked with the correct response, class, label, or known outcome per case and learns from that data to develop an algorithm to predict future outcomes on new unseen datasets. Supervised learning can be used for both classification (prediction of a dichotomous/binary/multilabel outcome) and regression (prediction of a continuous outcome; **Fig. 1**).
• Unsupervised learning: a subdivision of ML that uses raw, unlabeled data with no associated outcomes to identify naturally occurring patterns in the data that can be used to divide the data into subgroups. A common term for unsupervised learning is clustering (**Fig. 2**).
• Classification and regression tree (CART): a specific classification predictive model that enables the visualization of the rules set for an outcome prediction on other variables. Its output is a decision tree whereby each fork is split in a predictor variable and each end node contains a prediction for the outcome variable.
• Neural networks: a set of classification/regression algorithms modeled after the human brain, mimicking its complex structure of interacting nerves. A network contains layers of interconnected nodes. Each node applies an algorithm on the input to that node and then feeds the processed output to the next layer. Following a different number of layers, the output layer contains the final classification/prediction.
• Support vector machine (SVM): a set of supervised learning algorithms used for classification, regression, and outlier detection. SVM algorithms construct a hyperplane/set of hyperplanes in the data space to achieve maximal separation between data points.

[a] Department of Neurosurgery, Albany Medical College, 47 New Scotland Ave, Physicians Pavilion, 1st Floor, Albany, NY, 12208, USA; [b] Department of Neuroscience & Experimental Therapeutics, Albany Medical College, 47 New Scotland Ave, Albany, NY 12208, USA
* Corresponding author. AMC Neurosurgery Group, 47 New Scotland Ave, MC 10 Physicians Pavilion, 1st Floor, Albany, NY 12208.
E-mail address: jpilitsis@yahoo.com

Neurosurg Clin N Am 33 (2022) 351–358
https://doi.org/10.1016/j.nec.2022.02.012
1042-3680/22/© 2022 Elsevier Inc. All rights reserved.

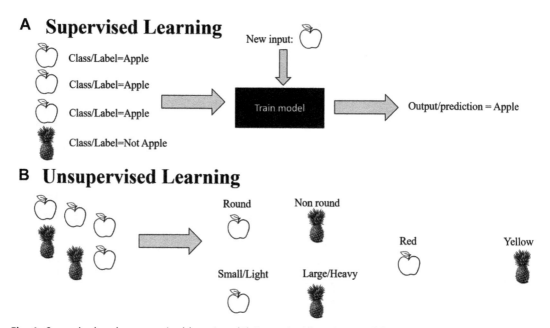

Fig. 1. Supervised and unsupervised learning. (*A*) Supervised learning models require labeled data (eg, apple/non-apple) to develop an algorithm that in turn classify a new unseen case (apple/non-apple). (*B*) Unsupervised learning can identify different patterns (size, color, weight, and so forth) and divide the data based on them. Not all patterns can be understandable by humans.

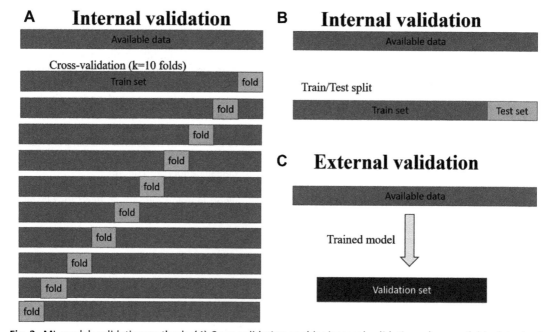

Fig. 2. ML models validation methods. (*A*) Cross-validation enables internal validation when available data size is limited. Data are split to k equal folds, and on each k iteration, the model trains on k-1 folds and tests performance on the k fold cases. The mean performance of k folds is considered generalizable. (*B*) Train/test split is the most common internal validation method, whereby the available data are split to train and test sets (usually at a 70/30 or 80/20 ratio). The model is then trained on the training set, and performance evaluated on the test set cases. (*C*) External validation can be performed once the model training has been complete. The trained model performance is tested on the cases in the unseen new external data.

- Train/test split: technique used to evaluate how the predictive performance of ML algorithms will generalize to an independent dataset. The dataset is split (eg, 70:30, 80:20) whereby the large portion is used to train the algorithm (train set), and the smaller portion is used to test the model predictions on these unseen samples (test set) (see **Fig. 2**).
- Cross-validation: resampling procedure used to evaluate how the predictive performance of ML models will generalize to an independent dataset on a limited sample (see **Fig. 2**).
- Feature: an input variable that is an individual measurable characteristic of a phenomenon being observed (eg, age, gender, pain location).
- Feature selection: the process of selecting a subset of the most valuable variables for model predictive performance from a set of data. Thus, features with a small effect on predictive performance will not be selected.
- Feature extraction: the process of building features from raw data by transforming primary features into new informative ones that can be used in ML models.

BACKGROUND

ML underlies many technologies commonly used in our daily lives. Examples include navigation applications' ability to estimate predicted time to a set location, targeted online advertising, suggested content through social media, identification of credit card fraud, and refinement of search engine results. Similarly, ML is rapidly integrating into many aspects of health care. ML-driven algorithms have been developed for diagnosis of diseases, radiological imaging diagnosis, new drugs discovery, and outcome prediction for improving management and treatment decisions.[1–5]

One study compared an ML-based model to the manual diagnosis by radiologists for 14 clinically important pathologies in chest radiographs. The ML model had similar diagnostic performance but at a rate of 1.5 minutes for 420 radiographs compared with 240 minutes for the radiologists.[6] In the surgical field, ML-driven algorithms for outcome prediction to modulate treatment have shown efficacy. Corey and colleagues[7] developed a model based on demographic and medical data from 88,000 encounters to determine postsurgical complications risk. The model achieved a positive predictive value of 35% in 12,000 subsequent encounters, meaning 1 in 3 patients identified by the algorithm suffered from a postsurgical complication within 30 days.[7]

Within the field of neurosurgery, ML-based models have been used to predict surgical outcomes in Cushing's disease with more than 80% performance[8] as well as lumbar stenosis with 54% to 80% performance,[9] among others. In a systematic review of artificial intelligence in neurosurgery, Sender and colleagues[10] demonstrated that ML algorithms outperformed clinical experts in 58% of measured outcomes, there was no difference in 36% of measured outcomes, and that the clinical experts outperformed ML algorithms in 6% of measured outcomes. Overall, these data suggest the important role of ML algorithms in augmenting decision-making and the predictive power of clinicians.

DISCUSSION
Clinical Utility of Machine Learning in Pain

ML derived algorithms serve as a promising means to refine patient selection for therapies by predicting outcomes to the treatment and identifying predictors of a positive response in an effort to improve overall outcomes. Within the realm of pain management, refined patient selection for more invasive procedures is paramount. Chronic pain is a common condition with a prevalence of up to 30.7% in the United States.[11] Patients who are refractory to medical treatment may be candidates for more invasive treatment including neuromodulation (spinal cord stimulation (SCS), dorsal root ganglion (DRG) stimulation, peripheral nerve stimulation (PNS)) and implantation of intrathecal drug delivery systems.

The success of these pain management interventions is largely dependent on appropriate patient selection. While these are successful in many patients, these invasive procedures do not provide pain relief to all patients and come at a significant financial cost with the risk of complication. Although several studies have demonstrated the cost-effectiveness of neuromodulation in appropriate patients compared with medical management,[12,13] removal of these devices due to nonresponse and ineffective pain relief reduce financial benefit. A removal rate of up to 10% to 15% has been documented in these devices.[14–16] Beyond cost and the potential for complication, poor patient selection delays other possible therapeutic interventions which may be more beneficial. Consequently, the optimization of patient selection is one of the most important aspects in improving outcomes of neuromodulation and intrathecal drug delivery systems in pain patients.

ML has also been used to identify phenotypes of pain that may correlate with outcome. The International Association for the Study of Pain defines it as "an unpleasant sensory and emotional experience associated with actual or potential tissue damage."[17] It is clinically evaluated using self-reported scales such as the numerical rating scale (NRS) or visual analog scale (VAS). While these subjective methods are considered the gold standard for measuring pain and quantifying the effectiveness of pain management therapies, the accuracy, and reliability of these measures are limited and can be affected by a series of immeasurable factors (eg, psychological, environmental). Furthermore, subjective measures are used to quantify the efficacy and define the outcomes of pain management therapies. Ultimately, ML offers an advanced technique to identify objectively measured features or phenotypes of pain that would allow for better assessment of pain outcomes.[18]

Machine Learning Algorithms to Improve Patient Selection

Supervised ML derived algorithms are being increasingly applied in pain management to define the phenotypes of patients who respond to specific therapies and create predictive models.[19–23] Two recent studies have offered preliminary work in predicting treatment response to neuromodulation therapies, specifically within SCS.[21,22] Despite the proven efficacy and growing use of SCS, failure rates are high and costly with no clear understanding of which patients benefit long-term, emphasizing the practicality of these predictive algorithms.

In one such study, De Jaeger and colleagues[21] developed a predictive model using CART in patients who had failed standard SCS and responded to high dose-SCS, a salvage waveform. They found that pain intensity scores, medication use, paresthesia coverage for back pain, and EQ5D for leg pain predicted response to high dose-SCS after 12 months.[21] Although these predictive features were identified, the model was not validated internally or externally. Internal validation in ML derived algorithms is critical to avoid overfitting of the data and low performance when applied on an external cohort.

In another recent study, Goudman and colleagues[22] used several ML-based algorithms to predict high frequency (HF)-SCS responders with a specificity and sensitivity of 90%. Selected variables included NRS, medication quantification scale III, age, and Oswestry Disability Index (ODI). Although it demonstrated high specificity and sensitivity, it did not achieve accuracy or overall predictive performance more than 58.33%.[22] Additionally, by splitting their 119 patients into train/test segments with 80% used to train the model and 20% used to test the model only one time (out of many possible random 20% splits), the model was not cross-validated and was prone to both over- and under-fitting.

Our research group also recently developed a predictive algorithm for long-term patient response to SCS placement with relatively high performance using methods that attempted to address the challenges encountered by other ML predictive outcome studies. We used the combination of unsupervised and supervised learning. We first used unsupervised ML techniques to identify subgroups, or clusters, within our dataset. Subsequently, supervised ML techniques were then applied to each distinct cluster to develop predictive algorithms for responders and high responders. In addition, we used nested cross-validation technique to validate our findings. Our predictive models demonstrated the highest overall performance with a predictive value of 70% to 75% success. This combined unsupervised-supervised learning approach yielded high predictive performance, suggesting that advanced ML derived approaches have the potential to be used as a functional clinical tool to improve long-term outcomes in SCS and other pain management devices.

Methodologic Considerations for Machine Learning to Improve Patient Selection

As described above, the combined methodology of unsupervised-supervised ML techniques is a promising method in pain outcome research (see **Fig. 1**). Although this combination of unsupervised and supervised learning has historically been used in the context of diagnostic image processing and fraud detection,[24,25] it is being increasingly applied to clinical medical data cohorts. Similarly, Elbattah and colleagues[26] demonstrated that the combined unsupervised-supervised approach provides higher predictive performance compared with the supervised classification alone in hip replacement surgery outcomes. To the best of our knowledge, this is the first use of this combined approach in this specific neuromodulation field and in pain research in general.

The cross-validation method is an important tool to avoid over-fitting a dataset and having low external validity—a weakness seen in many ML studies (see **Fig. 2**). This approach reduces the overfitting of data and the optimistic bias in error estimation in small sample sizes,[27,28] which is often the case in neuromodulation and pain studies. To adjust the algorithms and used features on small sample size, a nested cross-validation approach is required. Nested cross-

Nested cross validation

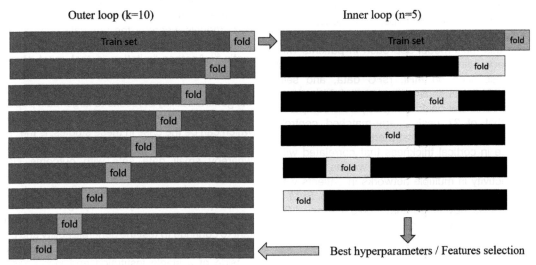

Fig. 3. Nested cross-validation. The nested cross-validation methods enable to optimize model hyperparameters and features selection when available data are limited. Data are split to k equal folds on the outer loop, whereby the model trains on k-1 folds and tests performance on the k fold cases. For each iteration/fold in the outer loop, that iteration train set is split again to n folds, whereby the model tests different hyperparameter sets and features on n-1 folds and tests them on n fold cases. The best hyperparameters and features in n folds of the inner loop are selected and then used for the evaluation of the k fold in the outer loop.

validation divides the data set into training and validation components through 2 separate loops (**Fig. 3**). In the outer loop, a dataset can be randomly divided into k (commonly k = 10) folds. This means that on each iteration, 90% of the data will be used to train the model, and 10% of the data will be set aside for validation. In the inner loop, which resides within the training set of the outer loop, the dataset can be split into n folds for hyperparameter tuning and feature selection. Hyperparameters refer to adjustable features that are fine-tuned to obtain a model with optimal performance. Feature selection refers to the process of reducing input variables to those that contribute most to prediction. Thus, the best hyperparameters and features selected in the inner loop are used to train on the training set and evaluated on the validation set of the external loop (see **Fig. 3**).

Several other methodologies that can improve ML techniques should be mentioned. Dimensionality reduction can be used to remove redundant or least important information in a dataset. Ensemble methods combine several prediction algorithms to get a higher quality prediction than what each model would have provided by itself. Commonly, a voting system between each predictive model is used to produce a final output (eg, if 2 out of 3 models classify a patient as a responder, it would produce a final prediction for a responder).

While ML shows strong potential in identifying pain subgroups using unsupervised learning, and developing predictive algorithms using supervised learning, methodology must be optimized to avoid potential pitfalls of ML that could affect the generalizability of the findings. The methodology for the development of ML algorithms is paramount to maximize the efficacy of its predictive power.

Machine Learning Techniques to Identify Biomarkers of Pain

In an effort to define an objective, measurable indicator of pain, prior studies have attempted to define physiologic and radiographic correlates of pain. For example, previous imaging studies have revealed certain cortical and subcortical areas are activated during the pain experience.[29,30] Electroencephalograph (EEG) data have demonstrated that spontaneous oscillations are suppressed in pain[31] and peak alpha frequency recorded at the temporal scalp correlates with pain severity.[32] Resting-state functional connectivity (rsFC) studies have also demonstrated alternations in neural connectivity that correlates the pain severity.[33,34] However, while these studies have added to our understanding of the brain mechanisms underlying pain, we still do not have a well-defined biomarker that can be reliably correlated with pain.[35] Consequently, multivariate ML techniques have been increasingly used in an attempt to identify features of pain and capture objective measures of the pain experience.

In a recent study, Lamichhane and colleagues[36] used this multi-modal approach in patients with low-back pain. Morphologic changes in cortical thickness seen on MRI, rsFC data, and self-reported clinical summary scores of 24 patients with chronic low-back pain (LBP) were compared with that of 27 healthy age-matched controls (HC). The results demonstrated a widespread difference in cortical thickness that correlated with the clinical summary scores, as well as increased connectivity in multiple networks in patients with LBP. Using the supervised ML technique, SVM, a model was developed that could classify LBP from HC subjects based on morphologic changes with an accuracy of 74.51%.

Another study by Fernandez Rojas and colleagues[37] used ML techniques to analyze functional near-infrared spectroscopy (FNIRS) data to identify a possible biomarker of pain. Pain information was collected from 18 volunteers using the thermal test of the quantitative sensory testing protocol. Feature extraction from time, frequency, and wavelet data were used to obtain 69 features. Feature selection was used to rank these features using various learning models, including SVM. It found that SVM could be used to identify pain with 94.17% accuracy with 25 features. It is important to note that these studies only assess pain as a dichotomous variable and do not quantify pain levels.

Taken a step further, ML derived markers of pain have been used to predict response to treatment. In an EEG study, Gram and colleagues[38] predicted the analgesic effect of morphine on tonic pain based on EEG data using SVM with an accuracy of 72%. Similarly, Lostch and colleagues[39] used supervised ML algorithms to construct a classifier based on a cold-water pain test that could predict the risk of persistent surgical pain after breast cancer surgery.

ML represents a powerful tool that will continue to advance our understanding of pain and pain management. Its ability to formulate patterns and classify large amount of data allows us to assess EEG, neuroimaging, rsFC, neural activity, and other forms of data in a meaningful way that objectifies pain into a quantitative measurement devoid of bias. Ultimately, the use of objectively measured biomarkers would enable improved accuracy in the assessment of pain outcomes and classification of responders and nonresponders to therapy. Perhaps in the future, pain management therapies will be guided based on the bio-derived pain signature of each patient.

Limitations of Machine Learning

There are limitations inherent to ML algorithms. These algorithms are often referred to as "black box" models whereby the rationale and calculations for the generated outputs remain enigmatic.[40] Another limitation is that most studies are single institution developed from a limited number of subjects, which may potentially limit the generalizability of results to larger pain populations. Another consequence of a small dataset, which can be the case in these studies, is the "accuracy paradox." This is a phenomenon of ML whereby small data sets with outcome class imbalance (eg, significantly more nonresponders than responders) can have an artificially high predictive performance by classifying all cases as nonresponders. Consequently, it remains important to continue to test the generalizability and predictive ability of these algorithms by expanding outside of a single institution and incorporating new external datasets into the model.

SUMMARY

ML-based techniques have numerous emerging applications that will have a profound influence on the future of pain medicine. By enabling large and complex data processing and learning, ML provides new tools that could change the current construct of pain management. These include the ability to objectify pain, identify pain phenotypes, and predict patients' outcomes to optimize appropriate selection for each treatment modality. Nevertheless, it should be stressed ML requires high-quality datasets and the methodological know-how for high-yield applications.

CONFLICT OF INTERESTS

Dr. Pilitsis is a consultant for Boston Scientific, Nevro, TerSera, and Abbott and receives grant support from Medtronic, Boston Scientific, Abbott, Nevro, TerSera, NIH 2R01CA166379-06 and NIH U44NS115111. She is medical advisor for Aim Medical Robotics and Karuna and has stock equity.

REFERENCES

1. Arcadu F, Benmansour F, Maunz A, et al. Deep learning algorithm predicts diabetic retinopathy progression in individual patients. NPJ Digital Med 2019;2:92.
2. Willemink MJ, Koszek WA, Hardell C, et al. Preparing medical imaging data for machine learning. Radiology 2020;295(1):4–15.

3. Karthik R, Menaka R, Johnson A, et al. Neuroimaging and deep learning for brain stroke detection - A review of recent advancements and future prospects. Comput Methods Programs Biomed 2020; 197:105728.

4. Vamathevan J, Clark D, Czodrowski P, et al. Applications of machine learning in drug discovery and development. Nat Rev Drug Discov 2019;18(6):463–77.

5. Heo J, Yoon JG, Park H, et al. Machine learning-based model for prediction of outcomes in acute stroke. Stroke 2019;50(5):1263–5.

6. Rajpurkar P, Irvin J, Ball RL, et al. Deep learning for chest radiograph diagnosis: a retrospective comparison of the CheXNeXt algorithm to practicing radiologists. PLoS Med 2018;15(11):e1002686.

7. Corey KM, Kashyap S, Lorenzi E, et al. Development and validation of machine learning models to identify high-risk surgical patients using automatically curated electronic health record data (Pythia): a retrospective, single-site study. PLoS Med 2018; 15(11):e1002701.

8. Zoli M, Staartjes VE, Guaraldi F, et al. Machine learning-based prediction of outcomes of the endoscopic endonasal approach in Cushing disease: is the future coming? Neurosurg Focus 2020;48(6):E5.

9. Siccoli A, de Wispelaere MP, Schröder ML, et al. Machine learning-based preoperative predictive analytics for lumbar spinal stenosis. Neurosurg Focus 2019;46(5):E5.

10. Senders JT, Arnaout O, Karhade AV, et al. Natural and artificial intelligence in neurosurgery: a systematic review. Neurosurgery 2018;83(2):181–92.

11. Johannes CB, Le TK, Zhou X, et al. The prevalence of chronic pain in United States adults: results of an Internet-based survey. J Pain 2010;11(11):1230–9.

12. Kumar K, Malik S, Demeria D. Treatment of chronic pain with spinal cord stimulation versus alternative therapies: cost-effectiveness analysis. Neurosurgery 2002;51(1):106–15 [discussion: 115-6].

13. Kumar K, Rizvi S. Cost-effectiveness of spinal cord stimulation therapy in management of chronic pain. Pain Med 2013;14(11):1631–49.

14. Negoita S, Duy PQ, Mahajan UV, et al. Timing and prevalence of revision and removal surgeries after spinal cord stimulator implantation. J Clin Neurosci 2019;62:80–2.

15. Brinzeu A, Cuny E, Fontaine D, et al. Spinal cord stimulation for chronic refractory pain: Long-term effectiveness and safety data from a multicentre registry. Eur J Pain 2019;23(5):1031–44.

16. Nissen M, Ikäheimo TM, Huttunen J, et al. Long-Term outcome of spinal cord stimulation in failed back surgery syndrome: 20 years of experience with 224 consecutive patients. Neurosurgery 2019;84(5):1011–8.

17. Pain terms: a list with definitions and notes on usage. Recommended by the IASP Subcommittee on Taxonomy. Pain 1979;6(3):249.

18. Levitt J, Edhi MM, Thorpe RV, et al. Pain phenotypes classified by machine learning using electroencephalography features. NeuroImage 2020;223: 117256.

19. Alexander J Jr, Edwards RA, Manca L, et al. Integrating machine learning with microsimulation to classify hypothetical, novel patients for predicting pregabalin treatment response based on observational and randomized data in patients with painful diabetic peripheral neuropathy. Pragmatic Observational Res 2019;10:67–76.

20. Azimi P, Benzel EC, Shahzadi S, et al. Use of artificial neural networks to predict surgical satisfaction in patients with lumbar spinal canal stenosis: clinical article. J Neurosurg Spine 2014;20(3):300–5.

21. De Jaeger M, Goudman L, Brouns R, et al. The long-term response to high-dose spinal cord stimulation in patients with failed back surgery syndrome after conversion from standard spinal cord stimulation: an effectiveness and prediction study. Neuromodulation 2020. https://doi.org/10.1111/ner.13138.

22. Goudman L, Van Buyten JP, De Smedt A, et al. Predicting the response of high frequency spinal cord stimulation in patients with failed back surgery syndrome: a retrospective study with machine learning techniques. J Clin Med 2020;9(12):4131.

23. Russo M, Verrills P, Santarelli D, et al. A novel composite metric for predicting patient satisfaction with spinal cord stimulation. Neuromodulation 2020; 23(5):687–97.

24. Aissaoui OEL, El Madani YELA, Oughdir L, et al. Combining supervised and unsupervised machine learning algorithms to predict the learners' learning styles. Proced Computer Sci 2019;148:87–96. https://doi.org/10.1016/j.procs.2019.01.012.

25. Gatidis S, Scharpf M, Martirosian P, et al. Combined unsupervised-supervised classification of multiparametric PET/MRI data: application to prostate cancer. NMR Biomed 2015;28(7):914–22.

26. Elbattah M, Molloy O. Clustering-Aided Approach for Predicting Patient Outcomes with Application to Elderly Healthcare in Ireland. 2017. In Workshops at the Thirty-First AAAI Conference on Artificial Intelligence 2017 Mar 21.

27. Vabalas A, Gowen E, Poliakoff E, et al. Machine learning algorithm validation with a limited sample size. PLoS One 2019;14(11):e0224365.

28. Varma S, Simon R. Bias in error estimation when using cross-validation for model selection. BMC Bioinformatics 2006;7:91.

29. Mouraux A, Iannetti GD. The search for pain biomarkers in the human brain. Brain 2018;141(12): 3290–307.

30. Duerden EG, Albanese MC. Localization of pain-related brain activation: a meta-analysis of neuroimaging data. Hum Brain Mapp 2013;34(1):109–49.

31. Peng W, Hu L, Zhang Z, et al. Changes of spontaneous oscillatory activity to tonic heat pain. PLoS One 2014;9(3):e91052.

32. Nir RR, Sinai A, Moont R, et al. Tonic pain and continuous EEG: prediction of subjective pain perception by alpha-1 power during stimulation and at rest. Clin Neurophysiol 2012;123(3):605–12.

33. Hemington KS, Wu Q, Kucyi A, et al. Abnormal cross-network functional connectivity in chronic pain and its association with clinical symptoms. Brain Struct Funct 2016;221(8):4203–19.

34. Cagnie B, Coppieters I, Denecker S, et al. Central sensitization in fibromyalgia? A systematic review on structural and functional brain MRI. Semin Arthritis Rheum 2014;44(1):68–75.

35. Levitt J, Saab CY. What does a pain 'biomarker' mean and can a machine be taught to measure pain? Neurosci Lett 2019;702:40–3.

36. Lamichhane B, Jayasekera D, Jakes R, et al. Multimodal biomarkers of low back pain: a machine learning approach. Neuroimage Clin 2021;29:102530.

37. Fernandez Rojas R, Huang X, Ou KL. A machine learning approach for the identification of a biomarker of human pain using fNIRS. Scientific Rep 2019;9(1):5645.

38. Gram M, Graversen C, Olesen AE, et al. Machine learning on encephalographic activity may predict opioid analgesia. Eur J pain (London, England) 2015;19(10):1552–61.

39. Lötsch J, Ultsch A, Kalso E. Prediction of persistent post-surgery pain by preoperative cold pain sensitivity: biomarker development with machine-learning-derived analysis. Br J Anaesth 2017;119(4):821–9.

40. Cabitza F, Rasoini R, Gensini GF. Unintended consequences of machine learning in medicine. JAMA 2017;318(6):517–8.